AF893196

Methods in Molecular Biology

Series Editor
John M. Walker
School of Life and Medical Sciences
University of Hertfordshire
Hatfield, Hertfordshire, AL10 9AB, UK

For further volumes:
http://www.springer.com/series/7651

Immune Checkpoint Blockade

Methods and Protocols

Edited by

Yago Pico de Coaña

Department of Oncology-Pathology, Karolinska Institutet, Stockholm, Sweden

Humana Press

Editor
Yago Pico de Coaña
Department of Oncology-Pathology
Karolinska Institutet
Stockholm, Sweden

ISSN 1064-3745 ISSN 1940-6029 (electronic)
Methods in Molecular Biology
ISBN 978-1-4939-8978-2 ISBN 978-1-4939-8979-9 (eBook)
https://doi.org/10.1007/978-1-4939-8979-9

Library of Congress Control Number: 2018965167

© Springer Science+Business Media, LLC, part of Springer Nature 2019
This work is subject to copyright. All rights are reserved by the Publisher, whether the whole or part of the material is concerned, specifically the rights of translation, reprinting, reuse of illustrations, recitation, broadcasting, reproduction on microfilms or in any other physical way, and transmission or information storage and retrieval, electronic adaptation, computer software, or by similar or dissimilar methodology now known or hereafter developed.
The use of general descriptive names, registered names, trademarks, service marks, etc. in this publication does not imply, even in the absence of a specific statement, that such names are exempt from the relevant protective laws and regulations and therefore free for general use.
The publisher, the authors, and the editors are safe to assume that the advice and information in this book are believed to be true and accurate at the date of publication. Neither the publisher nor the authors or the editors give a warranty, express or implied, with respect to the material contained herein or for any errors or omissions that may have been made. The publisher remains neutral with regard to jurisdictional claims in published maps and institutional affiliations.

This Humana Press imprint is published by the registered company Springer Science+Business Media, LLC, part of Springer Nature.
The registered company address is: 233 Spring Street, New York, NY 10013, U.S.A.

Preface

The immune system has a role in tumor surveillance and elimination that has been known for a long time, but not until recently have therapies been approved that make use of the full potential of the immune system to defeat cancer. Since the approval in 2011 of ipilimumab, an anti-CTLA-4 checkpoint blockade antibody, the interest in tumor immunology and immunotherapy has skyrocketed. In this volume of *Methods in Molecular Biology*, we aim to describe a series of techniques that are essential for evaluating the efficacy of new checkpoint blockade therapies as well as understanding the mechanisms behind the already approved ones.

There are several main focus points that can be addressed when studying antitumor immune responses. On the one hand, the basic elements to carry out the experiments should be readily available, such as purified T cells and patient-derived cancer cell lines. Additionally, complete information from the current status of the patients' immune system will generate the hypotheses that should be further tested in the lab with different functional assays. Finally, good in vivo animal models are essential to confirm the data obtained in vitro and close the bedside-bench-bedside circle of translational research. This book includes methodologies that provide the tools to cover these four focus points in the tumor immunology lab.

The first part consists of an approach to the characterization of the immune system on two levels: on the one hand, describing the tumor microenvironment can be essential for understanding its interactions with the immune system; on the other hand, the status of the immune system at a systemic level is also critical for understanding antitumor responses. This first part of the book includes microscopy techniques (Chapters 1 and 2) and techniques that describe via different approaches the type of immune cells that can be involved in the response (Chapters 3 and 4). In Chapter 5, the methodology for analyzing the immunopeptidome presented to T cells is shown. Finally, Chapter 6 provides the detailed protocol to analyze the abundance of microRNAs that are candidates to have an immunomodulatory function.

The main objective of the second part is to describe functional assays that provide answers to questions that may be raised after studying the immune system and its responses to immunotherapies. In order to have the possibility of carrying out these functional assays, both tumor-infiltrating lymphocytes (TIL) and tumor cell lines are needed; the detailed protocols on how to isolate and expand TIL and how to establish tumor cell lines are included in Chapters 7 and 8, respectively. This second part continues with different techniques that will evaluate the functional capacity of the main players of the antitumor immune response: T cells (Chapters 9 and 10) and NK cells (Chapters 11, 12, and 13).

Finally, the use of animal models is approached in the third part. Two different types of animal models are referenced: patient-derived xenograft models (Chapter 14) and the establishment of a syngeneic model (Chapter 15), followed by the analysis of tissue-resident cells in two different syngeneic models (Chapter 16).

The methods described in this volume not only apply to the understanding of checkpoint blockade, but they also are extremely useful in the study of tumor immunology and the development of new immunotherapies.

I would like to thank all contributors for their input and dedication. Their efforts have crystalized into a book that will be of great interest to the tumor immunologist. I would also like to thank the series editor, Professor John Walker, for giving me the opportunity to work on this project, offering guidance, dedication, and large doses of patience.

Stockholm, Sweden ***Yago Pico de Coaña***

Contents

Contributors

CARMEN BALLESTEROS-MERINO • *Robert W. Franz Cancer Center, Earle A. Chiles Research Institute, Providence Portland Medical Center, Portland, OR, USA*

MICHAL BASSANI-STERNBERG • *Ludwig Centre for Cancer Research, University of Lausanne, Epalinges, Switzerland; Department of Oncology, University Hospital of Lausanne (CHUV), Lausanne, Switzerland*

MARCUS BAUER • *Medical Faculty, Institute of Pathology, Martin Luther University Halle-Wittenberg, Halle (Saale), Germany*

DANIEL BETHMANN • *Medical Faculty, Institute of Pathology, Martin Luther University Halle-Wittenberg, Halle (Saale), Germany*

CARLO B. BIFULCO • *Robert W. Franz Cancer Center, Earle A. Chiles Research Institute, Providence Portland Medical Center, Portland, OR, USA*

PETTER BRODIN • *Science for Life Laboratory, Division of Clinical Paediatrics, Department of Women's and Children's Health, Karolinska Institutet, Stockholm, Sweden; Department of Newborn Medicine, Karolinska University Hospital, Stockholm, Sweden*

JEANNETTE CANY • *Laboratory Medicine, Department of Hematology, Radboudumc, Nijmegen, The Netherlands*

CHLOE CHONG • *Ludwig Centre for Cancer Research, University of Lausanne, Epalinges, Switzerland; Department of Oncology, University Hospital of Lausanne (CHUV), Lausanne, Switzerland*

NATALY CRUZ RODRÍGUEZ • *Cancer Biology Research Group, National Cancer Institute of Colombia, Bogotá, Colombia*

MONIKA EHNMAN • *Department of Oncology-Pathology, Karolinska Institutet, Stockholm, Sweden*

ZIPEI FENG • *Robert W. Franz Cancer Center, Earle A. Chiles Research Institute, Providence Portland Medical Center, Portland, OR, USA*

BERNARD A. FOX • *Robert W. Franz Cancer Center, Earle A. Chiles Research Institute, Providence Portland Medical Center, Portland, OR, USA; Department of Molecular Microbiology and Immunology, Oregon Health and Science University, Portland, OR, USA*

MICHAEL FRIEDRICH • *Institute for Medical Immunology, Martin-Luther-University Halle-Wittenberg, Halle, Germany*

FELIPE GALVEZ-CANCINO • *Laboratory of Gene Immunotherapy, Fundación Ciencia & Vida, Santiago, Chile*

FRÍÐA BJÖRK GUNNARSDÓTTIR • *Cancer Immunology, Department of Translational Medicine, Lund University, Malmö, Sweden; Department of Oncology-Pathology, Karolinska Institute, Stockholm, Sweden*

SHAWN M. JENSEN • *Robert W. Franz Cancer Center, Earle A. Chiles Research Institute, Providence Portland Medical Center, Portland, OR, USA*

PETER KAATZSCH • *Medical Faculty, Institute of Pathology, Martin Luther University Halle-Wittenberg, Halle (Saale), Germany*

ROLF KIESSLING • *Department of Oncology-Pathology, Karolinska Institute, Stockholm, Sweden*

TADEPALLY LAKSHMIKANTH • *Science for Life Laboratory, Division of Clinical Paediatrics, Department of Women's and Children's Health, Karolinska Institutet, Stockholm, Sweden*
MARIA-FILOTHEI LAZARIDOU • *Institute for Medical Immunology, Martin-Luther-University Halle-Wittenberg, Halle, Germany*
LINA WIK LEISS • *Department of Oncology-Pathology, Karolinska Institutet, Stockholm, Sweden; Neuro Clinic, Haukeland University Hospital, Bergen, Norway*
JOHANNA LINEROS • *Cancer Biology Research Group, National Cancer Institute of Colombia, Bogotá, Colombia*
ALVARO LLADSER • *Laboratory of Gene Immunotherapy, Fundación Ciencia & Vida, Santiago, Chile*
ERNESTO LOPEZ • *Laboratory of Gene Immunotherapy, Fundación Ciencia & Vida, Santiago, Chile*
TANJA LÖVGREN • *Department of Oncology-Pathology, Karolinska Institutet, Stockholm, Sweden; Department of Immunology, Genetics and Pathology, Uppsala University, Uppsala, Sweden*
ANDREAS LUNDQVIST • *Department of Oncology and Pathology, Karolinska Institutet, Stockholm, Sweden*
FABIO MARINO • *Ludwig Centre for Cancer Research, University of Lausanne, Epalinges, Switzerland; Department of Oncology, University Hospital of Lausanne (CHUV), Lausanne, Switzerland*
PATRICIA MARMOL • *Department of Cellular and Molecular Biology, Karolinska Institute, Stockholm, Sweden*
ALEXANDER MARTENS • *Department of Dermatology, University Medical Center Tübingen, Tübingen, Germany*
LINA MARÍA MARTÍNEZ • *Cancer Biology Research Group, National Cancer Institute of Colombia, Bogotá, Colombia*
CHIARA MASSA • *Institute of Medical Immunology, Martin Luther University Halle-Wittenberg, Halle (Saale), Germany*
JEROEN MELIEF • *Department of Oncology-Pathology, Karolinska Institute, Stockholm, Sweden*
ARTUR MEZHEYEUSKI • *Department of Immunology, Genetics and Pathology, Uppsala University, Uppsala, Sweden*
JUSTINE MICHAUX • *Ludwig Centre for Cancer Research, University of Lausanne, Epalinges, Switzerland; Department of Oncology, University Hospital of Lausanne (CHUV), Lausanne, Switzerland*
JEFFREY S. MILLER • *Division of Hematology, Oncology and Transplantation, Department of Medicine, University of Minnesota Masonic Cancer Center, Minneapolis, MN, USA*
PABLO MORENO-RUIZ • *Department of Oncology-Pathology, Karolinska Institutet, Stockholm, Sweden*
SHI YONG NEO • *Department of Oncology-Pathology, Karolinska Institute, Stockholm, Sweden*
AINE O'REILLY • *Department of Oncology-Pathology, Karolinska Institute, Stockholm, Sweden*
GRAHAM PAWELEC • *Department of Internal Medicine II, University Medical Center, Tübingen, Germany; Health Sciences North Research Institute of Canada, Sudbury, ON, Canada*
NIKOLAOS PAZAITIS • *Medical Faculty, Institute of Pathology, Martin Luther University Halle-Wittenberg, Halle (Saale), Germany*

Yago Pico de Coaña • *Department of Oncology-Pathology, Karolinska Institute, Stockholm, Sweden*

Carol Stefany Rodríguez • *Bachelor Project in Biology, Francisco José de Caldas District University, Bogotá, Colombia*

Josefa Antonia Rodríguez • *Cancer Biology Research Group, National Cancer Institute of Colombia, Bogotá, Colombia; Bachelor Project in Biology, Francisco José de Caldas District University, Bogotá, Colombia*

Dhifaf Sarhan • *Department of Microbiology, Tumor and Cell Biology, Karolinska Institutet, Karolinska University Hospital, Stockholm, Sweden*

Barbara Seliger • *Institute for Medical Immunology, Martin-Luther-University Halle-Wittenberg, Halle, Germany*

Christopher Shipp • *Department of Internal Medicine II, University Medical Center, Tübingen, Germany*

Andre Steven • *Institute of Medical Immunology, Martin Luther University Halle-Wittenberg, Halle (Saale), Germany*

Georgiana Toma • *Institute of Medical Immunology, Martin Luther University Halle-Wittenberg, Halle (Saale), Germany*

Uta Sandy Tretbar • *Institute for Medical Immunology, Martin-Luther-University Halle-Wittenberg, Halle, Germany*

Irene van der Haar Àvila • *Department of Oncology-Pathology, Karolinska Institute, Stockholm, Sweden; Division of Tumor Biology and Immunology (B3), NKI-AvL, Amsterdam, The Netherlands*

Claudia Wickenhauser • *Medical Faculty, Institute of Pathology, Martin Luther University Halle-Wittenberg, Halle (Saale), Germany*

Stina Wickström • *Department of Oncology-Pathology, Karolinska Institute, Stockholm, Sweden*

Kristina Witt • *Department of Oncology and Pathology, Karolinska Institutet, Stockholm, Sweden*

Part I

Generating Hypothesis

Chapter 1

Double Immunohistochemistry and Digital Image Analysis

Pablo Moreno-Ruiz, Lina Wik Leiss, Artur Mezheyeuski, and Monika Ehnman

Abstract

Immunohistochemistry (IHC) is a commonly used technique for protein detection in tissue sections. The method requires high-affinity antibodies that are specific for the target proteins of interest. More advanced IHC techniques have been developed to meet the need for simultaneous detection of more than one target protein in the same tissue section. This chapter provides general guidelines for double IHC staining of formalin-fixed, paraffin-embedded tissue sections. Chromogenic substrates are chosen based on their excellent contrast and compatibility with the subsequent digital image analysis.

Key words FFPE, Double immunohistochemistry, Antibody, Chromogenic substrate, Digital image analysis

1 Introduction

The immunohistochemistry (IHC) technique is well established both in routine clinical pathology testing and biomedical research, where proteins are often investigated for their prognostic and/or predictive potential in a given tumor type. For instance, epidermal growth factor receptor 2 (HER2) expression levels in breast cancer are determined by IHC in order to decide whether anti-HER2 therapy is appropriate for the patient [1]. Likewise, the presence of mutated isocitrate dehydrogenase 1 (IDH1), a mutation known to impact positively on survival in gliomas, is tested by IHC [2]. Thus, IHC is currently applied in cancer diagnostics, influencing the choice of treatment modality, and gives prognostic information to clinicians and patients.

IHC relies on the ability of antibodies to bind antigens with high affinity and specificity, as well as the possibility to conjugate antibodies to tracer molecules such as enzymes and fluorophores. These tracers allow for the visualization of the bound antigen by colorimetric reactions or fluorescence. IHC can be performed with single or multiple sets of antibodies, allowing for the detection of

Yago Pico de Coaña (ed.), *Immune Checkpoint Blockade: Methods and Protocols*, Methods in Molecular Biology, vol. 1913, https://doi.org/10.1007/978-1-4939-8979-9_1, © Springer Science+Business Media, LLC, part of Springer Nature 2019

more than one protein simultaneously. In fluorescence microscopy, the specimen is illuminated, and the fluorophores emit light that is detected at certain wavelengths. This technique is widely used for multiplexed staining and may also be the preferred method when the antigens of interest have an overlapping expression pattern. Multiplexing is more challenging using colorimetric detection, mainly because available substrates often have poor contrast and are difficult to separate, both with the human eye and with imaging equipment. However, as elaborated below, the use of certain two-color combinations that can be scored manually or by digital image analysis presents a powerful tool. By the analysis of large patient series, this technique can be used to establish tumor-specific patterns of protein expression, vessel morphology and quantity, stromal characteristics, and inter- and intratumoral heterogeneity of these characteristics [3–6].

Present literature on IHC is extensive, and instead of describing this technique per se, this chapter will exemplify how double IHC can be utilized to establish biomarker panels with prognostic or response-predictive value. Useful tips and tricks are also provided on how to achieve the best results with respect to histological preservation, antibody dilution, and visualization. Notably, protocol optimization is always required for each type of tissue and antibody combination.

2 Materials

All reagents are stored according to the manufacturer's instructions and prepared at room temperature prior to use. Only freshly prepared buffers should be used. Companies providing listed materials are stated in parenthesis in the following sections. Distilled water and analytical grade reagents are used for preparing all solutions unless indicated otherwise.

2.1 Deparaffinization, Rehydration, and Dehydration

1. Histo-Clear II clearing agent (National Diagnostics, Atlanta, Georgia, USA).
2. 99.5%, 95%, 70% ethanol.
3. Distilled water.
4. Ventilated hood.
5. Slide rack.
6. Plastic jars for slide racks.

2.2 Antigen Retrieval, Blocking, and Antigen Labeling

1. Decloaking NxGen Chamber™ (Biocare Medical, California, USA) for heat-induced epitope retrieval (HIER) [7, 8].
2. Tris/EDTA and/or antigen retrieval solution (Dako Denmark A/S): mix 25 ml of 10× solution with 225 ml distilled water for one canister with 24 slides.

3. Blocking buffer of choice: 2.5% normal horse serum, ready-to-use (Vector Laboratories, Burlingame, CA), (*see* **Note 1**).
4. Wash buffers: phosphate-buffered saline (PBS), pH 7.4 + 0.1% Tween20 (Sigma Aldrich®, Missouri, USA), (PBS-T); Tris-buffered saline (TBS) solution, pH 8 + 0.1% Tween20 (Sigma Aldrich®, Missouri, USA), (TBS-T); Tris–HCl buffer solution, pH 8.3.
5. Rocking table.
6. Hydrophobic PAP pen for immunostaining.
7. Primary antibody diluted in PBS + 0.1% Tween20 (BSA can be added).
8. Tubes/vials of proper size.
9. ImmPRESS™-AP Polymer Anti-Mouse IgG (Vector Laboratories, Burlingame, CA).

2.3 Substrate Incubation, Visualization, and Image Capture

1. Alkaline phosphatase substrate kits (Vector Laboratories, Burlingame, CA).
2. Distilled water.
3. Humid chamber (*see* **Note 2**).
4. Tubes/vials of proper size.
5. Coverslips of a size that covers the tissue section/s, e.g., 24 × 40 mm (Menzel).
6. Permanent mounting medium (compatible with clearing agent and substrates).
7. Ventilated hood or workbench.
8. Light microscope (with camera) and/or slide scanner.

2.4 Digital Images Analysis

1. ImageJ (an open-source software).
2. Computer system with Linux, Mac OS X, and Windows. Can be run on both 32-bit and 64-bit modes.
3. Microsoft excel (or analogous spreadsheet application) for data managing.

3 Methods

All procedures are carried out at room temperature unless indicated otherwise. Carefully follow guidelines for safety precautions and waste handling procedures. Do not allow the sections to dry at any step.

In the example provided below, the first primary antibody, raised in rabbit, targets a common marker for mesenchymal cells, platelet-derived growth factor receptor β, and is detected with an

Table 1
Solutions and incubation times used in the deparaffinization and rehydration steps

Solution	Incubation time
Histo-Clear II	5 min
Histo-Clear II	5 min
Histo-Clear II	5 min
99.5% Ethanol	5 min
99.5% Ethanol	5 min
95% Ethanol	5 min
95% Ethanol	5 min
70% Ethanol	5 min
Distilled water	5 min

alkaline phosphate-linked detection system and Vector Blue as chromogenic substrate. The other primary antibody, raised in mouse, targets the endothelial cell marker CD34 and is detected with an alkaline phosphate-linked detection system and Vector Red.

3.1 Deparaffinization and Rehydration of the Samples

Prepare samples by deparaffinization with a clearing agent and rehydration in a series of decreasing alcohol concentrations [9]. The slides are preferably kept well separated in a rack that can be easily submerged in plastic jars containing solutions according to Table 1 (*see* **Note 3**).

3.2 Labeling of the First Antigen (PDGFRβ)

1. Antigen retrieval: Prepare the decloaking chamber by adding 500 ml water. Place the rack with slides in a heat stable canister filled with EDTA or another appropriate high pH antigen retrieval buffer. Run an antigen retrieval program set to 110 °C for 5 min (*see* **Note 4**). Wait until the temperature is down to 80 °C before the lid is opened. Allow the slides to cool down by slowly replacing the buffer with PBS-T. A more detailed instruction is found in the manual of the decloaking chamber.
2. Wash slides in PBS-T for 3 $\times$ 5 min with or without gentle side-to-side agitation on a rocking table (*see* **Note 5**).
3. Widely encircle each tissue section with a hydrophobic barrier pen before adding appropriate amount of blocking solution. Alternatively, the cover slip method can be tried, where added volumes are kept to a minimum (*see* **Note 6**).
4. Incubate for 30 min in a humid chamber.

5. Tap off excess blocking solution and add the PDGFRβ-directed primary antibody (3169S (28E1), Cell Signaling Technology®, Inc., Europe) at a 1:100 dilution in PBS-T using a tube of appropriate size. 0.1% immunohistochemical grade bovine serum albumin can be used in the buffer to avoid adsorption of the antibody to the tube (*see* **Note 7**).
6. Incubate the slides overnight (o.n.) in a humid chamber at 4 °C.
7. Wash as in **step 2**.
8. Apply the ImmPRESS™-AP Polymer Anti-Rabbit IgG secondary antibody reagent (species specificity according to the primary antibody host). Incubate 30 min in a humid chamber.
9. Wash 3 × 5 min with TBS-T.
10. Wash 1 × 5 min with 100 mM Tris–HCl pH 8.3.
11. Prepare the substrate solution according to the Vector Blue Alkaline Phosphatase Substrate kit protocol immediately prior use. Cover the tissue sections with substrate dilution and incubate 5–20 min or until the stain intensity is sufficient (*see* **Note 8**).
12. Wash 2 × 5 min with PBS-T.

3.3 Labeling of the Second Antigen (CD34)

1. Place the rack with slides in the decloaking chamber canister again, this time prepared with pH 9 antigen retrieval buffer as recommended in the product sheet for CD34 Class II-clone QBend 10 (Dako Denmark A/S). Run a mild antigen retrieval program at 90 ° C for 5 min to ensure that unwanted background signals, derived from previously added antibody reagents, are not generated in the subsequent steps (*see* **Note 9**).
2. Repeat Subheading 3.2, **steps 2–5**.
3. Prepare the primary antibody in PBS-T at an optimized dilution for the tissue (1:50) and add to the slides.
4. Incubate for 1 h in a humid chamber (*see* **Note 10**).
5. Wash 3 × 5 min with PBS-T (*see* Subheading 3.2, **step 2**).
6. Apply the ImmPRESS™-AP Polymer Anti-Mouse IgG secondary antibody reagent (species specificity according to the host of the primary antibody) (*see* **Note 7**).
7. Incubate 30 min in a humid chamber.
8. Wash 3 × 5 min with TBS-T.
9. Wash 1 × 5 min with 100 mM Tris–HCl.
10. Follow the Vector Red Alkaline Phosphatase Substrate kit protocol in the same way as in Subheading 3.2, **step 11**, with the Vector Blue substrate kit.
11. Wash 2× with PBS-T for 5 min.

Table 2
Solutions and incubation times used in the dehydration process

Solution	Incubation time
70% Ethanol	2 min
95% Ethanol	2 min
99.5% Ethanol	2 min
Histo-Clear II	2 min

3.4 Dehydration and Mounting

1. Place the slides in a rack and dehydrate with increasing concentrations of ethanol followed by clearing agent as described in Table 2 (*see* **Note 11**).
2. Apply a drop of mounting medium close to the tissue section and slowly mount with a cover slip from that side to avoid bubbles.
3. Allow the mounting medium to fully cure (harden), in order to reach the specified refractive index, before imaging (*see* **Note 12**).

3.5 Slide Digitalization and Digital Image Analysis

The double-stained slides are preferably scanned in a digital pathology slide scanner, such as Aperio ScanScope AT using the ×20 objective. Produced images are normally in the .svs file format. Image revision requires appropriate software, for instance, Aperio ImageScope software (download from Aperio) or QuPath (https://qupath.github.io). In the software, the regions of interest (ROI) must be selected and saved in .tiff or .jpeg format. These ROI images will be used for further image analysis.

The image-processing algorithm (macro) was developed for the ImageJ software (http://rsb.info.nih.gov/ij).

1. The algorithm utilizes CD34 staining to identify vessels. It is used to determine vessel density and vessel diameter (Fig. 1a, b).
2. The perivascular area is defined as the region within a specified distance from the vessel. In each such perivascular area region, the intensity of PDGFRβ staining is measured separately (Fig. 1c).
3. Finally, PDGFRβ staining is also used to identify the tumor stroma: the fraction of total area positive for PDGFRβ. This area is defined as the regions with the intensity of the PDGFRβ above a preset background value. Small "negative" regions (with minimal linear dimension up to 11 micrometers or 20 square pixels) inside the "positive" areas are considered positive. To exclude potential artifact contamination, small regions (up to 15 square micrometers or 50 square pixels) are categorized as marker negative even when having the expression intensity above threshold (Fig. 1d).

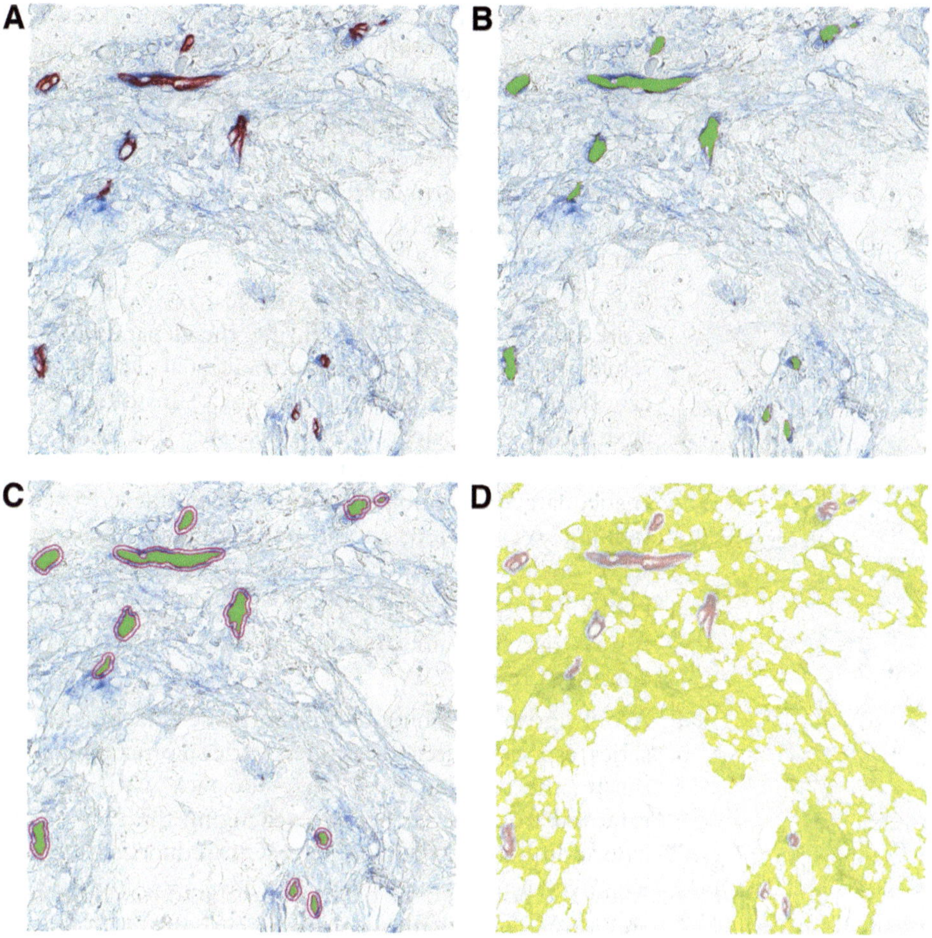

Fig. 1 Procedure for digital image analysis of vessel density. (**a**) Original image. Vessels are visualized by staining for CD34 (red), and pericytes/fibroblasts are visualized by staining for PDGFRβ (blue). (**b**) Apply automated green masks. Vascular elements are defined by digital image analysis. (**c**) Apply automated purple outlines. Perivascular regions are defined by image analysis. (**d**) Apply yellow overlay. Stroma regions are defined by image analysis

4. The stroma fraction is computed as the sum of all PDGFR-β-positive regions divided by the total ROI area. Average or median intensity of PDGFRβ expression in the stroma region can be quantified [Fig. 1 near here].

4 Notes

1. The blocking buffer is typically selected based on species compatibility with the secondary antibody reagents. In this protocol, the secondary antibodies originate from horse, and therefore, normal horse serum is a good choice to start with.

This step should however always be optimized, especially in tissues that are susceptible to high background staining.

2. A humid chamber is a tray that is designed to maintain a humid environment during all incubation steps to avoid evaporation from the slides. There are commercially available chambers for routine staining from different laboratory suppliers. Alternatively, a closed slide box with wet paper placed at the bottom can be used.
3. Wear gloves that meet your chemical protection needs and work in a ventilated hood during the deparaffinization and rehydration steps. Xylene is the traditional clearing agent but can be replaced with safer, less toxic, histological clearing agents that are biodegradable. Make sure that the sections are completely submerged in the solutions during the protocol. Inadequate deparaffinization may cause uneven background staining. All solutions should be exchanged regularly to preserve quality. To avoid unnecessary evaporation, always use plastic staining jars with lid.
4. Always use the same number of slide canisters per run for consistent results.
5. Avoid vigorous washing to prevent tissue detachment from the slides, especially after the antigen retrieval procedure. Similarly, during the washing steps, the slide rack with slides can be removed from the jar before exchanging the PBS-T solution. The addition of Tween20 (detergent) reduces surface tension.
6. Allow the bottom edge of the cover slip to touch the solution, and lower slowly, without trapping air bubbles.
7. Test different antibody dilutions to determine the optimal concentration for the tissue used. For example, if the manufacturer recommends a 1:100 dilution, make dilutions of at least 1:50, 1:100, and 1:200. Control for potential lot-specific variations in antibody concentration [10].
8. A white piece of paper can be placed under the slides to facilitate detection of the chromogenic substrate during development. Tap off the substrate solution and place the slide in a jar with Tris–HCl wash solution to hold further development. If needed, briefly check the blue color under the microscope (without allowing the sections to dry) to avoid a saturated signal. It is important to stop color development at the same time point for all sections if staining intensities are to be compared [11].
9. This step is particularly important if the two primary antibodies used are derived from the same species, and/or the secondary antibody-linked enzyme used for detection is the same for both antigens.

10. Many primary antibodies can be used at 4 °C o/n, or alternatively, at room temperature for 1 h.
11. Dehydration is not needed if a water-based mounting medium is used.
12. Always apply similar volumes of mounting medium in order to avoid variations in mounting quality between slides.

Acknowledgments

This work was supported by the Svenska Institutet to AM, the Swedish Childhood Cancer Fund (Barncancerfonden) and the Tornspiran Foundation (Stiftelsen Tornspiran) to ME, and the Knut and Alice Wallenberg Foundation to PM.

References

1. Perez EA, Cortés J, Gonzalez-Angulo AM, Bartlett JMS (2014) HER2 testing: current status and future directions. Cancer Treat Rev 40:276–284. https://doi.org/10.1016/j.ctrv.2013.09.001
2. Louis DN, Perry A, Reifenberger G et al (2016) The 2016 World Health Organization classification of tumors of the central nervous system: a summary. Acta Neuropathol 131:803–820. https://doi.org/10.1007/s00401-016-1545-1
3. Frödin M, Mezheyeuski A, Corvigno S et al (2016) Perivascular PDGFR-β is an independent marker for prognosis in renal cell carcinoma. Br J Cancer 116(2):195–201. https://doi.org/10.1038/bjc.2016.407
4. Mezheyeuski A, Bradic Lindh M, Kyrre Guren T et al (2014) Survival-associated heterogeneity of marker-defined perivascular cells in colorectal cancer. Oncotarget 7:41948–41958. https://doi.org/10.18632/oncotarget.9632
5. Corvigno S, Wisman GBA, Mezheyeuski A et al (2016) Markers of fibroblast-rich tumor stroma and perivascular cells in serous ovarian cancer: inter- and intra-patient heterogeneity and impact on survival. Oncotarget 7:18573–18584. https://doi.org/10.18632/oncotarget.7613
6. Corvigno S, Frödin M, Bea G et al (2017) Multi-parametric profiling of renal cell, colorectal, and ovarian cancer identifies tumour-type-specific stroma phenotypes and a novel vascular biomarker. J Pathol Clin Res 3:214–224. https://doi.org/10.1002/cjp2.74
7. Leong TY, Leong AS (2007) How does antigen retrieval work? Adv Anat Pathol 14:129–131. https://doi.org/10.1097/pap.0b013e31803250c7
8. Ramos-Vara JA (2017) Principles and methods of immunohistochemistry. Humana Press, New York, NY, pp 115–128
9. Boenisch T (2007) Pretreatment for immunohistochemical staining simplified. Appl Immunohistochem Mol Morphol 15:208–212. https://doi.org/10.1097/01.pai.0000209862.28205.e6
10. Smith A (2014) Finding the best antibody dilution by repeated immunostaining of the same tissue section. Biotech Histochem 89:215–219. https://doi.org/10.3109/10520295.2013.834074
11. Nguyen D, Nguyen D (2013) Quantifying chromogen intensity in immunohistochemistry via reciprocal intensity. Protoc Exch. https://doi.org/10.1038/protex.2013.097

Chapter 2

Multispectral Fluorescence Imaging Allows for Distinctive Topographic Assessment and Subclassification of Tumor-Infiltrating and Surrounding Immune Cells

Claudia Wickenhauser, Daniel Bethmann, Zipei Feng, Shawn M. Jensen, Carmen Ballesteros-Merino, Chiara Massa, Andre Steven, Marcus Bauer, Peter Kaatzsch, Nikolaos Pazaitis, Georgiana Toma, Carlo B. Bifulco, Bernard A. Fox, and Barbara Seliger

Abstract

Histomorphology has significantly changed over the last decades due to technological achievements in immunohistochemistry (IHC) for the visualization of specific proteins and in molecular pathology, particularly in the field of in situ hybridization of small oligonucleotides and amplification of DNA and RNA amplicons. With an increased availability of suitable methods, the demands regarding the observer of histomorphological slides were the supply of complex quantitative data as well as more information about protein expression and cell-cell interactions in tissue sections. Advances in fluorescence-based multiplexed IHC techniques, such as multispectral imaging (MSI), allow the quantification of multiple proteins at the same tissue section. In histopathology, it is a well-known technique for over a decade yet harboring serious problems concerning quantitative preciseness and tissue autofluorescence of multicolor staining when using formalin-fixed, paraffin-embedded (FFPE) tissue specimen. In recent years, milestones in tissue preparation, fluorescent dyes, hardware imaging, and software analysis were achieved including automated tissue segmentation (e.g., tumor vs. stroma) as well as in cellular and subcellular multiparameter analysis.

This chapter covers the role that MSI plays in anatomic pathology for the analysis of FFPE tissue sections, discusses the technical aspects of MSI, and provides a review of its application in the characterization of immune cell infiltrates and beyond regarding its prognostic and predictive value and its use for guidance of clinical decisions for immunotherapeutic strategies.

Key words Fluorescence microscopy, Multispectral imaging, Immune cells, Phenotyping

Claudia Wickenhauser, Daniel Bethmann, Zipei Feng and Shawn M. Jensen contributed equally to this work.

Yago Pico de Coaña (ed.), *Immune Checkpoint Blockade: Methods and Protocols*, Methods in Molecular Biology, vol. 1913,
https://doi.org/10.1007/978-1-4939-8979-9_2, © Springer Science+Business Media, LLC, part of Springer Nature 2019

1 Introduction

In recent years, it has become obvious that the role of the immune system in the modulation of malignancies is far more complex than originally anticipated. Although plenty of data indicate the importance of the innate and adaptive immune cells to control cancer progression, some immune cell subpopulations promote either directly or indirectly tumor growth and enhance survival of cancer cells, such as regulatory T cells (Tregs), myeloid-derived suppressor cells (MDSCs), and tumor-associated macrophages (TAM). An increasing body of evidence exists that tumor-infiltrating immune cells create different tumor microenvironments (TME) depending on their type and interaction. The presence, composition, and interactions between infiltrating immune cells, cancer cells, and stroma influence the induction and effector phase of anticancer immunity [1], can be linked to a better prognosis, and play an essential role in mediating the response to immunotherapy and affect clinical outcomes in many cancer subtypes.

Tumor cells express tumor antigens presented by human leukocyte antigens (HLA), which can be recognized by the host $CD8^+$ cytotoxic T lymphocytes (CTL). However, tumors often escape immune control by, e.g., downregulation or loss of HLA class I antigens and upregulation of co-inhibitory molecules. Furthermore, the local immune cell infiltrate undergoes dynamic alterations leading to an immune suppressive or immune stimulatory TME. This immune contexture is determined by the frequency, composition, functional state, and organization of the leukocyte infiltrate of the tumor and provides essential information relevant for prognosis, prediction of treatment response, and other pharmacodynamic parameters. Based on cellular and molecular characteristics of the TME, two categories of tumor escape exist. The first is characterized by a T cell-inflamed phenotype consisting of many infiltrating T cells, a broad chemokine profile, and a type I interferon (IFN) signature indicative for innate immune activation. These tumors can resist immune attack through dominant inhibitory effects of immune system-suppressive pathways. The second phenotype lacks the presence of T cells and resists immune attack through immune system exclusion or ignorance [2]. Colorectal cancer is a typical example, in which a correlation of immune classifications with molecular subclassifications has been described. The microsatellite instable-enriched subgroup characterized by overexpression of genes specific to cytotoxic lymphocytes has a good prognosis, while the microsatellite stable subgroup characterized by a high density of fibroblasts producing tumor-associated inflammation and supporting angiogenesis and by a low T cell infiltration has a poor prognosis [3]. In addition, in early-stage disease, the presence of activated $CD8^+$ CTL both within the tumor and in the peri-tumoral stroma had significant positive prognostic impact [4, 5]. The prognostic value of this immune phenotype might be even more powerful than the traditional staging [6, 7]. However, considering the complexity of possible interactions, it became clear that a proper evaluation of the TME requires much more information of a histological slide than just the data of CTL density. A methodologic platform offering evaluation of immune cell subsets and information concerning probability of cellular interactions has the potential to discover fundamental details of the tumor-host interaction.

So far, tissue microarrays (TMAs) have been commonly used as a powerful tool for the analysis of immune cell infiltrates and offer the opportunity to understand patient's disease condition, to improve prognostic evaluations, and to select the best treatment option [8, 9]. However, to address the high variability of tissue samples, parameters such as co-expression of molecules, spatial relationships between immune cells, heterogeneity, low abundance molecules, and other components of the TME, multiplex immunohistochemistry has to be employed [10]. This technology allows the exploration of the relationship between different cell types in the peri-tumoral and intratumoral compartments through more comprehensive and efficient analyses of the TME and the quantification of changes in the expression or state of specific biomarkers, which have an impact on patients' disease status. This will potentially advance the knowledge of immune phenotypes and cell interactions in the microenvironment and might provide an improved patient treatment based on individual TME responses to immunotherapy leading to enhanced response rates of tumor patients.

The development of a large panel of fluorophores with a broad spectral range allows simultaneous imaging of different cellular, subcellular, or molecular components, but the background staining is a major problem. In 2005, Lichtman and Conchello published a methodologic manual with the aim to describe concepts that underpin fluorescence microscopy and highlight some of the pitfalls frequently encountered [11]. Two years later Toth and Mezey illustrated possibilities to transfer the method for staining of FFPE slides [12]. With the technique of tyramide signal amplification, they realized multicolor staining of even rare and abundant antigens. However, it was just in 2014 with the availability of new fluorophores and complex imaging software solutions that MSI was possible [13]. Since then, the commercial availability of suitable imaging platforms allowed the analyses of the TME in human tumors and their correlation with clinical parameters. Recently, a number of researchers and clinicians have used this novel technology for the characterization of the TME of different human tumor entities but also experimental murine models [14–17]. Most importantly it was possible to demonstrate for the first time that MSI allowed discriminating a subset of high-stage oral squamous

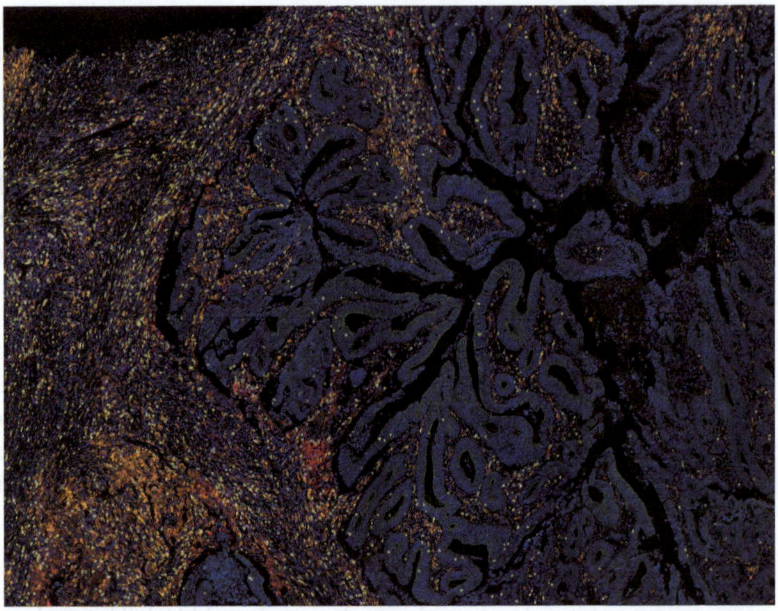

Fig. 1 Multiplex immunohistochemistry of colon cancer. Multispectral imaging was performed according to the protocol provided in this chapter. Shown are four images stitched together. CD3, magenta; CD8, yellow; CD163, orange; FoxP3, green; PD, L1, red; cytokeratin, cyan; DAPI, blue

cell carcinoma (OSCC) with favorable outcome [18]. It could also be illustrated that MSI is a suitable tool to predict the success of adoptive T cell transfer with expanded tumor-infiltrating lymphocytes in the context of malignant melanoma [19]. The application of this method has recently been further extended to proteins of signal transduction pathways that could be used as diagnostic or prognostic biomarkers to conduct tumor therapy [20]. This article provides the materials and a detailed experimental protocol used for multiplex IHC staining of human and murine tissues. Representative stainings using this method are shown for a colon carcinoma lesion (Fig. 1) and the murine B16F10 tumor model (Fig. 2).

2 Materials

2.1 Slide Preparation

1. For human studies: formalin-fixed, paraffin-embedded (FFPE) tissue samples (*see* Subheading 3.1.1).
2. For murine studies: zinc-fixed, paraffin-embedded tissue samples (*see* Subheading 3.2.1).
3. Superfrost Plus (charged) tissue slides.
4. Microtome.
5. Slide storage box.
6. Tissue floatation bath.

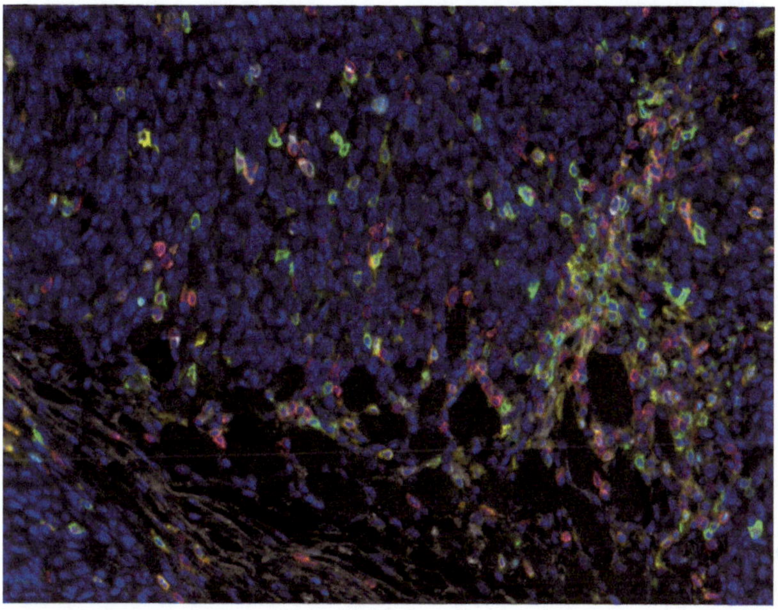

Fig. 2 Multispectral image of a murine B16F10 tumor. B16F10 melanoma tumor was analyzed by multiplex immunohistochemistry using the protocol described in this chapter. A representative image is shown. aCD3, red; CD4, yellow; CD8, green; FoxP3, cyan; GranzymeB, white; DAPI, blue

2.1.1 Formalin Fixation

1. 4.5% phosphate-buffered formalin.
2. Paraffin 50–52°.
3. Tissue cassettes.

2.1.2 Zinc Fixation

1. Zinc fixative: 0.5 g calcium acetate, 5.0 g zinc acetate, 5.0 g zinc chloride, 1000 mL 0.1 M Tris buffer at pH 7.4, mix to dissolve, the final pH will be approximately pH 6.5–7.0, and store at RT.
2. 70% ethanol.
3. Paraffin 50–52°.
4. Tissue cassettes.

2.2 Deparaffinization and Antigen Retrieval

1. Tissue Autostainer.
2. Xylenes.
3. 100% ethanol.
4. 10% neutral buffered formalin (NBF).
5. Slide staining dishes and racks.
6. Antigen retrieval pH 6.0 and pH 9.0 buffers (for human tissue only, included in Opal™ 7-color Manual IHC Kit, *see* below).
7. 1250 W microwave with inverter technology.

Table 1
Opal™ fluorophore excitation and emission maxima

Fluorophore	Channel	Excitation	Emission
Spectral DAPI	DAPI	358 nm	461 nm
Opal 520	FITC	494 nm	525 nm
Opal 540	FITC + Cy3	523 nm	536 nm
Opal 570	Cy3	550 nm	570 nm
Opal 620	Cy3 + Texas Red	588 nm	616 nm
Opal 650	Texas Red	627 nm	650 nm
Opal 690	Cy5	676 nm	694 nm

2.3 Antibody Staining: 7-Plex "Immune Cell" Panel (PD-L1, CD8, FoxP3, CD3, CD163, Cytokeratin, DAPI) for Human Tissues

1. Orbital Shaker.
2. StainTray™ 30 Place with Black Lid (Newcomer Supply).
3. ImmEdge™ Hydrophobic Barrier Pen (Vector Labs).
4. 5% H_2O_2: dilute from 30% H_2O_2 with double-distilled peroxidase-free H_2O (ddH_2O).
5. Rabbit antihuman-PD-L1 antibody (Cell Signaling Technology, clone E1L3N).
6. Rabbit antihuman-CD8 antibody (Spring Biosciences, clone SP239).
7. Mouse antihuman-FoxP3 antibody (Abcam, clone 236A/E7).
8. Rabbit antihuman-CD3 antibody (Spring Biosciences, clone SP7).
9. Prediluted mouse antihuman-CD163 antibody (Ventana, clone MRQ-26).
10. Mouse antihuman-cytokeratin antibody (Dako, clone AE1/AE3).
11. Opal™ 7-color Manual IHC Kit 50 slides (Perkin Elmer), containing:
    (a) Six fluorophores (Opal 520, Opal 540, Opal 570, Opal 620, Opal 650, Opal 690, *see* Table 1).
    (b) Spectral 4′,6-diamidin-2-phenylindol (DAPI).
    (c) 1× Plus Amplification Diluent.
    (d) Blocking/antibody diluent.
    (e) Opal Polymer HRP mouse + rabbit.
    (f) 10× antigen retrieval pH 6.0 buffer: dilute to 1× using ddH_2O.
    (g) 10× antigen retrieval pH 9.0 buffer: dilute to 1× using ddH_2O.

12. Alternatively use different PerkinElmer Opal™ Kits (e.g., "Tumor-Infiltrating Lymphocyte Kit"), including alternate sets of primary antibodies with respective preparation protocols.
13. Dimethyl sulfoxide (DMSO).
14. 1× Tris-buffered saline with Tween 20 (TBS-T): 10× TBS: 24.2 g Trizma Base (=25 nM), 80.0 g NaCl (=150 mM), 1000 mL autoclaved ddH_2O, mix to dissolve, adjust to pH 7.6 using HCl, in order to prepare 1000 mL of TBS-T add 100 mL 10× TBS to 900 mL dH_2O, then add 0.5 mL Tween-20™ (=0.05%), mix to dissolve, and store at room temperature (RT).
15. VectaShield™ Hardset Mounting Medium (Vector Labs).
16. Fast-drying nail polish.
17. Vacuum source.

2.4 Antibody Staining: 6-Plex "Immune Cell" Panel (CD3, CD19, CD8, CD4, F4/80, DAPI) for Murine Tissues

1. Orbital shaker.
2. StainTray™ 30 Place with Black Lid (Newcomer Supply).
3. ImmEdge™ Hydrophobic Barrier Pen (Vector Labs).
4. PeroxAbolish™ (Biocare Medical).
5. ImmPRESS™ HRP anti-rat IgG, mouse-adsorbed (peroxidase) polymer detection kit with goat serum (Vector Labs).
6. Renaissance™ Background Reducing Diluent (Biocare Medical).
7. Anti-rabbit HRP Polymer Conjugate (Thermo Fisher).
8. Rodent Decloaker™ (Biocare Medical).
9. Rabbit anti-mouse-CD3 antibody (Spring Bioscience, clone SP7).
10. Rat anti-mouse-CD19 antibody (BD Pharmingen, clone 1D3).
11. Rat anti-mouse-CD8 antibody (eBioscience, clone 4SM15).
12. Rat anti-mouse-CD4 antibody (eBioscience, clone 4SM95).
13. Rat anti-mouse-F4/80 antibody (AbD Serotec, clone Cl:A3-1).
14. Opal™ 7-color Manual IHC Kit 50 slides, containing:
    (a) Six fluorophores (Opal 520, Opal 540, Opal 570, Opal 620, Opal 650, Opal 690, *see* Table 1).
    (b) Spectral DAPI.
    (c) 1× Plus Amplification Diluent (# FP1498).
15. DMSO.
16. 1× TBS-T.

17. VectaShield™ Hardset Mounting Medium (Vector Labs).
18. Fast drying nail polish.
19. Vacuum source.

2.5 Imaging, Spectral Library, and Software Analysis

1. Vectra™ or Polaris™ Automated Quantitative Pathology Imaging System and Software (PerkinElmer).
2. Phenochart™ Software v.1.0.5 (Perkin Elmer).
3. InForm™ Image Analysis Software v.3.0.4 (Perkin Elmer).

3 Methods

3.1 Human Tissues: 7-Plex "Immune Cell" Panel (PD-L1, CD8, FoxP3, CD3, CD163, Cytokeratin, DAPI)

3.1.1 Formalin Fixation

1. Depending on tissue size/density, incubate tissue with formalin for 12–48 h.
2. Dehydrate fixed tissue.
3. Heat tissue and penetrate with soluble paraffin.
4. Mold a paraffin tissue block by cooling.
5. Store at RT.

3.1.2 Slide Preparation

1. Retrieve FFPE tissue blocks from pathology/laboratory.
2. Pre-chill samples on ice for 10 min and heat up water bath to 40 °C.
3. Slice 4 μM thick sections using the microtome and float sections onto Superfrost slides.
4. Place slides in storage box and let them dry at RT overnight.
5. Store slides at 4 °C until use.

3.1.3 Deparaffinization and Antigen Retrieval (1 Day Prior to Staining Procedure)

1. Prepare a maximum of 24 slides per run:
   (a) Eight control slides for each tissue type (seven single-plex slides to build the spectral library: Opal 520, Opal 540, Opal 570, Opal 620, Opal 650, Opal 690, DAPI plus 1 unstained slide to assess autofluorescence).
   (b) Up to 16 test slides; mark slides accordingly.
2. Heat slides in a dry oven at 55–60 °C for 1 h, positioned to allow drainage of melting paraffin, to strengthen tissue adhesion on slides.
3. Place slides onto staining rack in the Leica Autostainer and run deparaffinization protocol. Alternatively, wash slides by the hand in xylene 3× for 10 min and then hydrate through an ethanol gradient (5–10 min in 100% followed by 75, 50, 25%), ending in a water bath.
4. Refix tissue in NBF for 20 min followed by a water bath.

5. Mark the border of the tissue samples with a hydrophobic pen and let the slides dry for 5 min.
6. Place all the slides (control + test) in the staining rack.
7. Rinse the slides once with ddH_2O and immerse the slides in 1× antigen retrieval *pH 6.0* buffer.
8. Place the lid on the staining rack and then heat it in the microwave for approximately 1 min at 100% power (until it just reaches rolling boil), followed by 15 min on 10% power. Let the dish cool overnight.

3.1.4 Antibody Staining

First epitope: PD-L1

1. Place all test slides + one control slide (*Opal 650*) into a staining rack containing H_2O and rinse once. Leave the remaining slides in the "microwave" rack, lid on, at 4 °C until further usage.
2. Wash slides once with 1× TBS-T.
3. Withdraw each slide individually from the rack and vacuum off fluids, especially within the marked area, followed by placing the slides on the StainTray.
4. Block the slides using approximately 100 μL 1× blocking diluent for 10 min (the more the better), shaking at 100 rpm (*see* **Notes 1** and **2**).
5. Dilute *anti-PD-L1* primary antibody in 1× antibody diluent at a 1:200 concentration and add approximately 100 μL/slide, covering the whole tissue area. Incubate for 30 min at RT shaking at 100 rpm.
6. Vacuum off the primary antibody and wash the slides 3× 30 s in 1× TBS-T.
7. Add Opal™ Polymer HRP secondary antibody dropwise to cover the tissue area and incubate for 10 min at RT and 100 rpm.
8. Vacuum off the secondary antibody and wash the slides 3× 30 s in 1× TBS-T.
9. Dissolve *TSA-Opal 650* from Opal™ 7-color IHC kit in 150 μL DMSO, dilute 1:100 in 1× Plus Amplification Diluent, and add approximately 100 μL/slide to cover the tissue area. Incubate for 10 min at RT and 100 rpm (*see* **Note 3**). Store stock solution at 4 °C.
10. Vacuum off TSA and wash the slides 3× 30 s in 1× TBS-T.
11. Immerse all test + control slides in 1× antigen retrieval *pH 6.0* buffer.

12. Place the lid on staining rack and heat the dish in the microwave for 1 min on 100% power, followed by 10 min on 10% power. Let the dish cool for at least 15 min.
13. Repeat **steps 1–12** for the remaining five epitopes using these specific settings:

    CD8:

(a) Use all test slides plus one control slide (*Opal 570*).

(b) Dilute *anti-CD8* primary antibody in 1x antibody diluent at a 1:50 concentration; add approximately 100 μL/slide, covering the whole tissue area; and incubate for 45 min at RT shaking at 100 rpm.

(c) Dissolve *TSA-Opal 570* from Opal™ 7-color IHC kit in 150 μL DMSO, dilute 1:100 in 1× Plus Amplification Diluent, add approximately 100 μL/slide to cover the tissue area, incubate for 10 min at RT and 100 rpm, and store stock solution at 4 °C.

(d) Immerse all test + control slides in 1× antigen retrieval *pH 9.0* buffer.

FoxP3:

(a) Use all test slides plus one control slide (*Opal 520*).

(b) Dilute *anti-FoxP3* primary antibody in 1x antibody diluent at a 1:100 concentration; add approximately 100 μL/slide, covering the whole tissue area; and incubate for 45 min at RT shaking at 100 rpm.

(c) Dissolve *TSA-Opal 520* from Opal™™ 7-color IHC kit in 150 μL DMSO, dilute 1:100 in 1× Plus Amplification Diluent, add approximately 100 μL/slide to cover the tissue area, incubate for 10 min at RT and 100 rpm, and store stock solution at 4 °C.

(d) Immerse all test + control slides in 1× antigen retrieval *pH 6.0* buffer.

CD3:

(a) Use all test slides plus one control slide (*Opal 540*).

(b) Dilute *anti-CD3* primary antibody in 1× antibody diluent at a 1:50 concentration; add approximately 100 μL/slide, covering the whole tissue area; and incubate for 45 min at RT shaking at 100 rpm.

(c) Dissolve *TSA-Opal 540* from Opal™ 7-color IHC kit in 150 μL DMSO, dilute 1:100 in 1× Plus Amplification Diluent, add approximately 100 μL/slide to cover the tissue area, incubate for 10 min at RT and 100 rpm, and store stock solution at 4 °C.

(d) Immerse all test + control slides in 1× antigen retrieval *pH 6.0* buffer.

CD163:

(a) Use all test slides plus one control slide (*Opal 690*).

(b) Use prediluted *anti-CD163* primary antibody; add approximately 100 μL/slide, covering the whole tissue area; and incubate for 45 min at RT shaking at 100 rpm.

(c) Dissolve *TSA-Opal 690* from Opal™ 7-color IHC kit in 150 μL DMSO, dilute 1:100 in 1× Plus Amplification Diluent, add approximately 100 μL/slide to cover the tissue area, incubate for 10 min at RT and 100 rpm, and store stock solution at 4 °C.

(d) Immerse all test + control slides in 1× antigen retrieval *pH 6.0* buffer.

Cytokeratin:

(a) Use all test slides plus one control slide (*Opal 620*).

(b) Dilute *anti-cytokeratin* primary antibody in 1× antibody diluent at a 1:50 concentration; add approximately 100 μL/slide, covering the whole tissue area; and incubate for 45 min at RT shaking at 100 rpm.

(c) Dissolve *TSA-Opal 620* from Opal™ 7-color IHC kit in 150 μL DMSO, dilute 1:100 in 1× Plus Amplification Diluent, add approximately 100 μL/slide to cover the tissue area, incubate for 10 min at RT and 100 rpm, and store stock solution at 4 °C.

(d) Vacuum off TSA and wash the slides 3× 30 s in 1× TBS-T.

(e) Do not proceed to microwave step (**step 12**)!

3.1.5 DAPI Staining, Mounting, and Coverslip

1. Collect all test and control slides in the same rack containing TBS-T.
2. Dilute three droplets of spectral DAPI in 1 mL of ddH_2O; add approximately 100 μL/slide, covering the whole tissue area. Incubate for 5 min at RT and 100 rpm and store stock solution at 4 °C.
3. Vacuum off DAPI stain.
4. Wash the slides 2× 30 s in 1× TBS-T.
5. Rinse the slides once with H_2O and then let them dry at RT.
6. Coverslip the slides with Vectra Shield™ Hard Mount (*see* **Note 4**).
7. Paint the edge of the slide with nail polish to preserve slide.
8. Let the slides harden out at RT for 15–30 min.
9. Proceed to image acquisition or store slides at 4 °C in a covered slide box.

3.2 Murine Tissues: 6-Plex "Immune Cell" Panel (CD3, CD19, CD8, CD4, F4/80, DAPI)

3.2.1 Zinc Fixation

1. Depending on tissue size/density, incubate tissue with zinc fixative for 24–48 h.
2. Incubate tissue with 70% ethanol for 7 days.
3. Dehydrate fixed tissue.
4. Heat tissue and penetrate with soluble paraffin.
5. Mold a paraffin tissue block by cooling.
6. Store at RT.

3.2.2 Slide Preparation

1. Retrieve zinc-fixed, paraffin-embedded tissue blocks from the laboratory.
2. Pre-chill samples on ice for 10 min and heat up water bath to 40 °C.
3. Slice 4 μM thick sections using the microtome and float sections onto Superfrost slides.
4. Place slides in the storage box and let them dry at RT overnight (*see* **Note 5**).
5. Store slides at 4 °C until use.

3.2.3 Deparaffinization and Antigen Retrieval (1 Day Prior to the Staining Procedure)

1. Prepare a maximum of 24 slides per run:
   (a) Seven control slides for each tissue type (six single-plex slides to build the spectral library: Opal 520, Opal 540, Opal 570, Opal 650, Opal 690, DAPI plus 1 unstained slide to assess autofluorescence)
   (b) Up to 17 test slides; mark slides accordingly.
2. Place slides onto staining rack in the Leica Autostainer and run deparaffinization protocol. Alternatively, wash slides by the hand in xylene for 3× 10 min, followed by hydration through an ethanol gradient (5–10 min in 100%, then 70, 50, 25%), ending in a water bath.
3. Mark the border of the tissue sample with a hydrophobic pen and let the slides dry for 5 min (*see* **Note 6**).

3.2.4 Antibody Staining

First and second epitope: CD3, CD19

1. Place all test slides plus one control slide (*Opal 690*) in a staining rack containing 1× TBS-T. Leave the remaining slides in another rack containing 1× TBS-T, lid on, at 4 °C until further usage.
2. Withdraw each slide individually from the rack and vacuum off fluids, especially within marked area, followed by placing the slides on the StainTray.
3. Add 100 μL (50–200 μL depending on tissue size) of Perox-Abolish™ on tissue section within the marked tissue border.

Incubate for 30 min to block endogenous peroxidase (*see* **Note 2**).

4. Vacuum off PeroxAbolish.
5. Wash the slides once for 30 s with H_2O.
6. Wash the slides once for 30 s with 1× TBS-T.
7. Block the slides using approximately 100 μL goat serum for 30 min, shaking at 100 rpm.
8. Vacuum off goat serum.
9. Dilute *anti-CD3* primary antibody in Renaissance™ Background Reducing Diluent at 1:100 concentration; add approximately 100 μL/slide, covering the whole tissue area; and incubate for 40 min at RT shaking at 100 rpm.
10. Vacuum off the primary antibody.
11. Wash the slides 3× 30 s in 1× TBS-T.
12. Add approximately 100 μL of anti-rabbit HRP polymer conjugate/slide, covering the whole tissue area. Incubate for 15 min at RT shaking at 100 rpm.
13. Vacuum off the HRP polymer conjugate.
14. Wash the slides 3× 30 s in 1× TBS-T.
15. Dissolve *TSA-Opal 690* from Opal™ 7-color IHC Kit in 150 μL DMSO, dilute 1:100 in 1× Plus Amplification Diluent, add approximately 100 μL/slide to cover the tissue area, incubate for 10 min at RT and 100 rpm (*see* **Note 3**), and store stock solution at 4 °C.
16. Vacuum off TSA.
17. Wash the slides 3× 30 s with 1× TBS-T.
18. Wash the slides once for 30 s with H_2O.
19. Extract *Opal 690* control slide from rack, replacing it with the *Opal 520* control slide.
20. Add approximately 100 μL of PeroxAbolish™ on tissue section within the marked tissue border. Incubate for 30 min.
21. Vacuum off PeroxAbolish™.
22. Wash the slides once for 30 s with H_2O.
23. Wash the slides once for 30 s with 1× TBS-T.
24. Block the slides using approximately 100 μL goat serum for 30 min, shaking at 100 rpm.
25. Dilute *anti-CD19* primary antibody in Renaissance™ Background Reducing Diluent at 1:100 concentration and add approximately 100 μL/slide, covering the whole tissue area. Incubate for 40 min at RT shaking at 100 rpm.
26. Vacuum off the primary antibody.

27. Wash the slides 3× 30 s in 1× TBS-T.
28. Add approximately 100 μL of ImmPRESS™ anti-rat HRP secondary antibody/slide, covering the whole tissue area. Incubate for 15 min at RT shaking at 100 rpm.
29. Vacuum off the secondary antibody.
30. Wash the slides 3× 30 s with 1× TBS-T.
31. Dissolve *TSA-Opal 520* from Opal™ 7-color IHC Kit in 150 μL DMSO, dilute 1:100 in 1× Plus Amplification Diluent, add approximately 100 μL/slide to cover the tissue area, incubate for 10 min at RT and 100 rpm, and store stock solution at 4 °C.
32. Vacuum off TSA.
33. Wash the slides 3× 30 s with 1× TBS-T.
34. Wash the slides once for 30 s with H_2O.
35. Immerse all test + control slides in Rodent Decloaker™.
36. Place the lid and heat the dish in the microwave for approximately 1 min on 100% power (until it just reaches rolling boil), followed by 10 min on 10% power.
37. Let the dish cool to RT.
38. Wash the slides once for 30 s with H_2O.
39. Wash the slides once for 30 s with 1× TBS-T.

Third to fifth epitope: CD8, CD4, F4/80

40. Repeat **steps 20–39** for the remaining three epitopes, using these specific settings:

CD8:

(a) Use all test slides plus 1 control slide (*Opal 570*).
(b) Dilute *anti-CD8* primary antibody in Renaissance™ Background Reducing Diluent at 1:100 concentration; add approximately 100 μL/slide, covering the whole tissue area; and incubate for 40 min at RT shaking at 100 rpm.
(c) Add approximately 100 μL of ImmPRESS™ anti-rat HRP secondary antibody/slide, covering the whole tissue area. Incubate for 15 min at RT shaking at 100 rpm.
(d) Dissolve *TSA-Opal 570* from Opal™ 7-color IHC Kit in 150 μL DMSO, dilute 1:100 in 1× Plus Amplification Diluent, add approximately 100 μL/slide to cover the tissue area, incubate for 10 min at RT and 100 rpm, and store stock solution at 4 °C.
(e) Immerse all test + control slides in Rodent Decloaker™, followed by the microwave step.

CD4:

(a) Use all test slides + 1 control slide (*Opal 540*).

(b) Dilute *anti-CD4* primary antibody in Renaissance™ Background Reducing Diluent at 1:100 concentration and add approximately 100 μL/slide, covering the whole tissue area. Incubate for 40 min at RT shaking at 100 rpm.

(c) Add approximately 100 μL of ImmPRESS™ anti-rat HRP secondary antibody/slide, covering the whole tissue area. Incubate for 15 min at RT shaking at 100 rpm.

(d) Dissolve *TSA-Opal 540* from Opal™ 7-color IHC Kit in 150 μL DMSO, dilute 1:100 in 1× Plus Amplification Diluent, add approximately 100 μL/slide to cover the tissue area, incubate for 10 min at RT and 100 rpm, and store stock solution at 4 °C.

(e) Immerse all test + control slides in Rodent Decloaker™, followed by the microwave step.

F4/80:

(a) Use all test slides plus 1 control slide (*Opal 650*).

(b) Dilute *anti-F4/80* primary antibody in Renaissance™ Background Reducing Diluent at 1:100 concentration and add approximately 100 μL/slide, covering the whole tissue area. Incubate for 40 min at RT shaking at 100 rpm.

(c) Add approximately 100 μL of ImmPRESS™ anti-rat HRP secondary antibody per slide, covering the whole tissue area, and incubate for 15 min at RT shaking at 100 rpm.

(d) Dissolve *TSA-Opal 650* from Opal™ 7-color IHC Kit in 150 μL DMSO, dilute 1:100 in 1× Plus Amplification Diluent, add approximately 100 μL/slide to cover the tissue area, incubate for 10 min at RT and 100 rpm, and store stock solution at 4 °C.

(e) Vacuum off TSA and wash the slides 3× 30 s in 1× TBS-T.

(f) Do not proceed to microwave step (**step 36**)!

3.2.5 DAPI Staining, Mounting, and Coverslip

1. Collect all test and control slides in the same rack, containing TBS-T.
2. Dilute three droplets of spectral DAPI in 1 mL of ddH_2O and add approximately 100 μL/slide, covering the whole tissue area. Incubate for 5 min at RT and 100 rpm. Store stock solution at 4 °C.
3. Vacuum off DAPI stain.
4. Wash the slides 3× 30 s in 1× TBS-T.
5. Rinse the slides once with H_2O and then let them dry at RT.

6. Coverslip the slides with VectaShield™ Hard Mount (*see* **Note 4**).
7. Paint the edge of the slide with nail polish to preserve slide.
8. Let the slides harden out at RT for 15–30 min.
9. Proceed to image acquisition or store slides at 4 °C in a covered slide box.

3.3 Imaging, Spectral Library, and Software Analysis (Identical in Human and Murine Specimen)

1. Open Vectra™/Polaris™ software and insert control slides in the microscope as per manual instructions.
2. Create images for setup of *spectral library* (one for each tissue type) as per manual instruction at 200× resolution using the seven (six for murine tissue) single-plex control slides (Opal 520, Opal 540, Opal 570, Opal 620, Opal 650, Opal 690, DAPI). Assess exposure times for each fluorophore individually and only in the channels as provided in Table 1 while setting a "generic" exposure time of 150 ms for all the remaining channels.
3. Open InForm™ software to build and manage spectral library as per manual instructions.
4. Insert test slides plus the autofluorescence control slide in the microscope.
5. Create a new protocol.
6. Select a representative region of interest (ROI) on the tissue slide with sizable epitope prevalence (*see* **Note** 7). (Auto-) Focus tissue samples.
7. Assess exposure times for all channels at 100× and 200× resolution while preventing overexposure (red dots/areas). In general the shorter the exposure times and the smaller the range between all exposure times, the better while still collecting a specific signal. Try to generate exposure times of DAPI vs. the other fluorophores at a ratio of no more than 1:4.
8. Save protocol.
9. Scan test slides as per manual instructions at 100x resolution, using a specific label and the saved protocol.
10. Scan autofluorescence control slide using the same protocol.
11. Open Phenochart™ software.
12. Review 100× image. Select 3–5 (or more) representative ROIs for 20× MSI imaging, e.g., covering both the tumor's invasive margin (IM) and core (CT).
13. Use Vectra™/Polaris™ software to scan slides at 20× resolution as per manual instructions creating multilayered "IM3" files.
14. Open InForm™ software. To utilize *batch analysis*, open 1–3 representative IM3 files of each test-plus the autofluorescent

control slide. Alternatively select and continue with all IM3 files of the test plus the autofluorescent control slide.

15. Unmix channels using the specific spectral library created in **step 3** for the selected tissue.
16. Use autofluorescence control slide to extract tissue autofluorescence as per manual instructions.
17. Exercise specific epitope labels and balance epitope intensity as per manual instructions.
18. Run tissue segmentation (e.g., selecting tumoral and stromal compartment, *see* **Note** 7), cell segmentation (assessing cell membrane, cytoplasm, and nucleus compartment), and phenotyping (as well as scoring if applicable) as per manual instructions. Make sure to completely finish each step before continuing to the next step, as changing settings in a prior step will erase all progress from this step onward. Make sure to save each step of the way in an InForm™ project/protocol file.
19. Batch-analyze all IM3 files of the test slides using InForm's "batch analysis" mode, utilizing the previously saved settings to the whole cohort.
20. Merge and process data in Excel™ and R™. Perform relevant statistical analysis in SPSS™ or Prism™.

4 Notes

1. When processing human tissues with high endogenous peroxidase activity and/or elevated amounts of erythrocytes, additional treatment might improve the results: before the first blocking step (**step 4**), add 100 μL of 5% H_2O_2 solution on tissue section within the marked tissue border, and incubate for 30 min at RT, shaking at 100 rpm, to quench endogenous peroxidase.
2. When processing multiple slides, take into account the time it takes between adding solution to the first slide and the last slide (i.e., if it takes 2 min to add reagents to all slides, incubate for additional 8 min).
3. When adding TSA-Opal reagents on the tissue, do not exceed an incubation time of 10 min as the background can significantly increase.
4. Do not use mounting medium containing DAPI as this will significantly increase the background.
5. When processing murine tissues, do not heat slides for tissue adhesion as this will damage the epitopes.

6. When processing murine tissues, no antigen retrieval is required.
7. In some cases, the cytokeratin antibody cocktail (AE1/AE3) might not completely stain all tumor/epithelial cells. For tissue segmentation to separate tumor from stroma, it is important to include (if applicable) plenty of sample images from tumors that are negative for the cocktail as well as to include DAPI in the segmentation training.

Acknowledgments

Claudia Wickenhauser, Daniel Bethmann, Zipei Feng, and Shawn M. Jensen contributed equally to this work.

References

1. Engels B, Engelhard VH, Sidney J et al (2013) Relapse or eradication of cancer is predicted by peptide-major histocompatibility complex affinity. Cancer Cell 23(4):516–526
2. Gajewski TF, Schreiber H, Fu Y-X (2013) Innate and adaptive immune cells in the tumor microenvironment. Nat Immunol 14 (10):1014–1022
3. Becht E, de Reyniès A, Giraldo NA et al (2016) Immune and stromal classification of colorectal cancer is associated with molecular subtypes and relevant for precision immunotherapy. Clin Cancer Res 22(12):4057–4066
4. Pages F, Berger A, Camus M et al (2005) Effector memory T cells, early metastasis, and survival in colorectal cancer. N Engl J Med 353 (14):2654–2666
5. Galon J, Costes A, Sanchez-Cabo F et al (2006) Type, density, and location of immune cells within human colorectal tumors predict clinical outcome. Science 313(11):1960–1964
6. Mlecnik B, Tosolini M, Kirilovsky A et al (2011) Histopathologic-based prognostic factors of colorectal cancers are associated with the state of the local immune reaction. J Clin Oncol 29(7):610–618
7. Galon J, Pagès F, Marincola FM et al (2012) Cancer classification using the immunoscore: a worldwide task force. J Transl Med 10:205. https://doi.org/10.1186/s12967-017-1310-9
8. Abel EJ, Bauman TM, Weiker M et al (2014) Analysis and validation of tissue biomarkers for renal cell carcinoma using automated high-throughput evaluation of protein expression. Hum Pathol 45(5):1092–1099
9. van Zwieten A (2013) Tissue microarray technology and findings for diagnostic immunohistochemistry. Pathology 45(1):71–79
10. Gorris MAJ, Halilovic A, Rabold K et al (2018) Eight-color multiplex immunohistochemistry for simultaneous detection of multiple immune checkpoint molecules within the tumor microenvironment. J Immunol 200(17):347–354
11. Lichtman JW, Conchello JA (2005) Fluorescence microscopy. Nat Methods 2 (12):910–919
12. Toth ZE, Mezey E (2007) Simultaneous visualization of multiple antigens with tyramide signal amplification using antibodies from the same species. J Histochem Cytochem 55 (6):545–554
13. Stack EC, Wang C, Roman KA et al (2014) Multiplexed immunohistochemistry, imaging, and quantitation: a review, with an assessment of Tyramide signal amplification, multispectral imaging and multiplex analysis. Methods 70 (1):46–58
14. Mezheyeuski A, Bergsland CH, Backman M et al (2018) Multispectral imaging for quantitative and compartment-specific immune infiltrates reveals distinct immune profiles that classify lung cancer patients. J Pathol 244 (4):421–431. https://doi.org/10.1002/path.5026
15. Ying L, Yan F, Meng Q et al (2017) Understanding immune phenotypes in human gastric disease tissues by multiplexed immunohistochemistry. J Transl Med 15:206–210. https://doi.org/10.1186/s12967-017-1311-8
16. Feng Z, Shawn M, Jensen SM et al (2016) Multispectral Imaging of T and B Cells in

Murine Spleen and Tumor. J Immunol 198 (4):3943–3950

17. Ng SSM, Nagy BA, Jensen SM et al (2017) Heterodimeric IL15 treatment enhances tumor infiltration, persistence, and effector functions of adoptively transferred tumor-specific T cells in the absence of lymphodepletion. Clin Cancer Res 23(17):2817–2830
18. Feng Z, Puri S, Moudgil T et al (2015) Multispectral imaging of formalin-fixed tissue predicts ability to generate tumor-infiltrating lymphocytes from melanoma. J Immunother Cancer 3:47. https://doi.org/10.1186/s40425-015-0091-z
19. Feng Z, Bethmann D, Kappler M et al (2017) Multiparametric immune profiling in HPV-oral squamous cell cancer. JCI Insight 2 (14):1–17
20. Yang L, Liu Z, Tan J et al (2018) Multispectral imaging reveals hyper active TGF-β signaling in colorectal cancer. Cancer Biol Ther 19 (2):105–112

Chapter 3

Systems-Level Immune Monitoring by Mass Cytometry

Tadepally Lakshmikanth and Petter Brodin

Abstract

As therapies involving the modulation, stimulation, and deliberate excitation of the immune system are becoming routine, better methods for monitoring immune responses in human patients are needed. Mass cytometry allows for detailed profiling of all immune cell populations and their functional responses using a simple blood sample. When combined with appropriate computational analyses, the resolution for distinguishing desired responses from unproductive or even adverse reactions to immunotherapeutic interventions increases. Here we describe a core experimental and computational framework for global, systems-level immune monitoring by mass cytometry.

Key words Mass cytometry, Systems immunology, CyTOF, Human immunology, Tumor immunology, Immune monitoring

1 Introduction

Mass cytometry or cytometry by time-of-flight (CyTOF™, Fluidigm Inc.) is a method developed by Scott Tanner and colleagues at the University of Toronto in order to increase the number of simultaneous protein measurements in individual cells, over what was previously possible using state-of-the-art flow cytometry [1]. This was achieved by coupling antibodies to polymer backbones containing chelator groups preloaded with rare earth metal ions, each with a unique mass, providing a unique mass tag for each antibody. Cells stained with such antibodies can then be analyzed individually using a ICP-MS-type instrument, for single-cell sample introduction and analysis. The first high-level demonstration using this technology revealed a global analysis of human bone marrow samples that reconstructed the entire hematopoietic tree of cell differentiation [2]. Following this landmark study, a number of groups have revealed the utility of mass cytometry for describing human immune system variation [3, 4], immune cell variation among tissues [5], identification of rare antigen-specific cells [6], and immune cells infiltrating tumor tissue [7, 8]. Recently this

Yago Pico de Coaña (ed.), *Immune Checkpoint Blockade: Methods and Protocols*, Methods in Molecular Biology, vol. 1913, https://doi.org/10.1007/978-1-4939-8979-9_3,

© Springer Science+Business Media, LLC, part of Springer Nature 2019 method has been applied to patients undergoing immunotherapy of cancer and revealed differences associated with clinical outcome [9], and novel mechanisms of action for checkpoint inhibitors [10].

2 Materials

2.1 Reagents

1. RPMI complete medium: RPMI-1640, 10% FBS, 1% penicillin–streptomycin, L-glutamine (from 100× supplement).
2. RPMI-ICS medium: RPMI-1640, 2% FBS, 1% penicillin--streptomycin, L-glutamine (from 100× supplement).
3. Thawing medium: RPMI-1640, 10% FBS, 1% penicillin–streptomycin, L-glutamine, 25 U/ml Benzonase® Nuclease (from 2.5×10^5 U/ml stock).
4. Frozen-thawed human peripheral blood mononuclear cells (PBMCs) or freshly isolated PBMCs. For sample type processing details, refer to Subheadings 3.1.1 and 3.1.2, respectively.
5. 0.4% trypan blue.
6. 0.5 M EDTA: use 2 mM final concentration.
7. CyFACS buffer: 1× PBS, 0.1% BSA (from 30% stock), 2 mM EDTA (from 0.5 M stock), 0.05% Na-azide (from 10% stock). This buffer should be stored in LDPE bottles (*see* **Note 1**).
8. Metal-free 10× PBS (Rockland Immunochemicals): make 1× final concentration with Milli-Q grade water, and store in LDPE bottles.
9. Lymphoprep™ (STEMCELL Technologies).
10. SepMate™ −15 and −50 tubes (STEMCELL Technologies).
11. MaxPar metal-conjugated antibodies (Fluidigm).
12. MaxPar X8 polymer multimetal reaction kit (Fluidigm).
13. In-house coupled antibodies: 100 μg of a purified antibody is coupled per reaction (as per manufacturer's recommendations) (*see* **Note 2**).
14. Antibody stabilizer (CANDOR Bioscience GmbH).
15. Live–dead stain: Maleimide-DOTA loaded with 103Rh, 5 mg/ml (Macrocyclics, Inc.).
16. 5 mg/ml Brefeldin A: dissolved in dimethyl sulfoxide (DMSO) and frozen in small aliquots at −80 °C: *see* Table 2 for concentrations.
17. 1000× Golgi stop/Monensin (BioLegend): *see* Table 2 for concentrations.
18. Phorbol 12-myristate 13-acetate (PMA): *see* Table 1 for concentrations.
19. Ionomycin: *see* Table 1 for concentrations.

Table 1
Stimulating agents

Reagent	Stock concentration	Intermediate dilution (concentration)	Final concentration
Phorbol 12-myristate 13-acetate (PMA)	1 mg/ml (in DMSO)	1:1000 of stock (0.001 mg/ml) in RPMI-ICS	1:100 of intermediate stock (10 ng/ml)
Ionomycin	1 mg/ml (in DMSO)	1:10 of stock (0.1 mg/ml) in RPMI-ICS	1:100 of intermediate stock (1 μg/ml)
PHA	1 mg/ml (in sterile PBS)	–	5 μg/ml (200 μl for 40-ml medium)
LPS	0.1 mg/ml	1:10 of stock (0.01 mg/ml) in RPMI-ICS	1:20 of intermediate stock (0.5 μg/ml)
Anti-CD3 (immobilized)	0.5 mg/ml	–	10 μg/ml
Anti-CD28 (soluble)	0.5 mg/ml	–	5 μg/ml

Table 2
Protein secretion inhibitors

Reagent	Stock concentration	Intermediate dilution (concentration)	Final concentration
Brefeldin A (BFA)	5 mg/ml	1:10 of stock (0.5 mg/ml) in RPMI-ICS	1:100 of intermediate stock (5 μg/ml)
Golgi stop/monensin	1000×	1:10 of stock (100×) in RPMI-ICS	1:100 of intermediate stock (1×)

20. Anti-CD3, clones OKT3 or UCHT1 (BioLegend): *see* Table 1 for concentrations.
21. Anti-CD28, clone CD28.1 (BioLegend): *see* Table 1 for concentrations.
22. Phytohaemagglutinin (PHA): *see* Table 1 for concentrations.
23. Lipopolysaccharide (LPS): *see* Table 1 for concentrations.
24. Fc Receptor (FcR) blocking buffer (Cytodelics AB).
25. Cell-ID 20-Plex Pd Barcoding Kit (Fluidigm).
26. DMSO.
27. Intracellular fixation & permeabilization buffer set (eBioscience): Freshly make this buffer by mixing diluent and fix concentrate (1:4).
28. 10× saponin-based permeabilization buffer (eBioscience): 10× buffer diluted to 1× in Milli-Q water.

29. 16% paraformaldehyde (Polysciences, Inc.).
30. EQ™ four element calibration beads (Fluidigm).
31. 125 μM Cell-ID™ Intercalator-Ir (Fluidigm).
32. Milli-Q water.

2.2 Equipment and Supplies

1. Centrifuge with adaptors for 5-ml, 15-ml, and 50-ml tubes.
2. Water bath at 37 °C.
3. 37 °C humidified incubator with CO_2.
4. Laminar airflow (LAF) hood.
5. Nanodrop 2000 (Thermo Fisher Scientific).
6. Multiwell plates: 96-well U-bottom plates, 96-well deep-well 2-ml plates.
7. Dual-chamber counting slides (Bio-Rad).
8. Pipettors: calibrated single channel and multichannel.
9. ThawSTAR® CFT2 thawing instrument (BioCision).
10. TC20™ automated cell counter (Bio-Rad).
11. CyTOF® 2 mass cytometer (Fluidigm).
12. Cell strainers (70 μM).
13. Digital scale.
14. Round-bottom polystyrene tubes with cell strainer caps, 5-ml.
15. 15- and 50-ml falcon tubes.
16. 5-ml Eppendorf Tubes.
17. Sonicator.
18. Mr. Frosty™ freezing container (Nalgene).

3 Methods (*See* Fig. 1)

3.1 Sample Processing

3.1.1 Thawing and Resting PBMCs (See **Note 3**)

1. Pre-warm RPMI complete medium using 37 °C water bath. Each sample will need 20 ml of medium for thawing. Depending on the number of PBMC samples that are to be thawed, transfer the corresponding amount of pre-warmed RPMI complete medium to a separate tube, and to this, add Benzonase (1:10000; final concentration at 25 U/ml), thus called "thawing medium". Benzonase helps in preventing cell clumping.
2. Remove samples from liquid nitrogen or −80 °C freezer, and transport to the lab using ThawSTAR CFT2 Transporter (BioCision) containing some dry ice.
3. Transfer 10 ml of thawing medium into a 15-ml falcon tube. Use one falcon tube per sample.
4. Thaw frozen cryovials using ThawSTAR® CFT2 thawing instrument (BioCision) with one sample thawed each time.

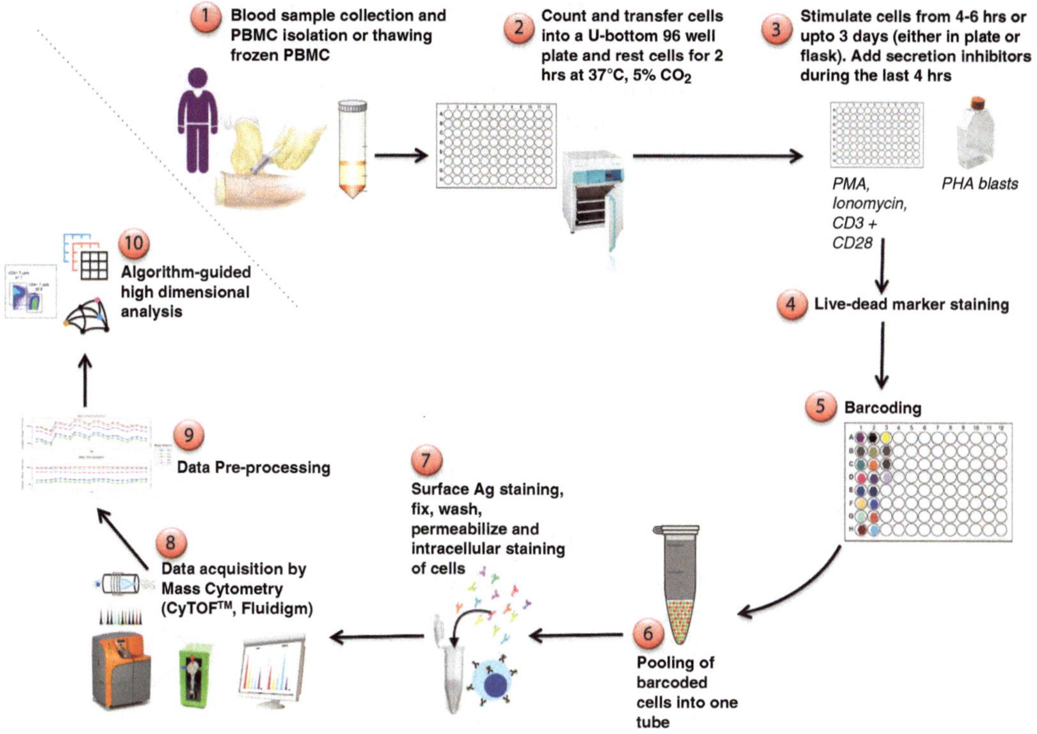

Fig. 1 Schematic of ICS assay workflow for systems-level immune monitoring by mass cytometry

ThawSTAR instrument (*see* **Note 4**) is placed in a biosafety cabinet before thawing and is turned on a few min prior to placing a cryovial in it.

5. When cells are thawed (*see* **Note 5**) as determined by ThawSTAR® instrument, add 1 ml of pre-warmed thawing medium from appropriately labeled falcon tube slowly to the cells and then transfer the cells to the falcon tube. Rinse vial with more medium to retrieve all of the cells, and transfer to the falcon tube.
6. Continue with the rest of the samples as quickly as possible (*see* **Note 6**).
7. Centrifuge cells at 300 × *g* for 10 min at room temperature.
8. Aspirate the supernatant, being careful to leave the pellet intact, gently tap the tube and resuspend in 10 ml of pre-warmed thawing medium again.
9. Centrifuge cells at 300 × *g* for 5 min at room temperature.
10. Aspirate supernatant, agitate the cell pellet by tapping the tube, and add 3 ml of pre-warmed RPMI-ICS medium (with no Benzonase from this step onward).
11. Count cells with TC20™ automated cell counter. To count, take 10 μl of cells and dilute with 10 μl of trypan blue [11], in

an empty V-bottom 96-well plate. Load onto a cell counting dual-chamber slide (Bio-Rad) with a 1:2 dilution factor.

12. Adjust the cell concentration to 10 × 10^6 cells/ml with pre-warmed RPMI-ICS medium (*see* **Note** 7), and add 200 μl with 2 × 10^6 cells/well or maximum available (if less than 2 × 10^6 cells/well) into each well of a U-bottom 96-well plate.
13. Each sample can be split equally into two or more wells keeping one as an unstimulated control and the other for stimulation.
14. Rest the cells for 2–4 h (*see* **Note 8**) at 37 °C in a CO_2 incubator.

3.1.2 Isolation of fresh PBMCs from Whole Blood or Buffy Coat (See Note 9)

1. PBMCs were isolated using Lymphoprep™ (STEMCELL Technologies) and SepMate™ 15 or 50 (STEMCELL Technologies) (*see* **Note 10**) as per the manufacturer's recommendations.
2. Count cells with TC20™ automated cell counter. To count, take 10 μl of cells and dilute with 10 μl of PBS in an empty V-bottom 96-well plate. Load onto a cell counting dual-chamber slide (Bio-Rad) with a 1:2 dilution factor.
3. Adjust the cell concentration to 10 × 10^6 cells/ml with pre-warmed RPMI-ICS medium, and add 200 μl with 2 × 10^6 cells or maximum available (if less than 2 × 10^6 cells/well) into each well of a U-bottom 96-well plate.
4. Each sample can be split equally into two or more wells keeping one as an unstimulated control and the other for stimulation.
5. No resting is needed for freshly isolated PBMCs.

3.1.3 Stimulating Cells

1. As mentioned above, two different cell types can be used for ICS assay:
   (a) Rested cells if cryopreserved PBMCs were thawed (*see* Subheading 3.1.1).
   (b) Freshly isolated PBMCs (*see* Subheading 3.1.2).
2. To cells (in 200 μl) transferred into each well of a U-bottom 96-well plate, add the activation reagents (with the exception of unstimulated control) for stimulation as directed in Table 1. Stimulate cells with different activation reagents as follows:
   (a) PMA and ionomycin: To cells in 200 μl/well with 2 × 10^6 cells in a U-bottom 96-well plate, add these reagents as directed in Table 1, and incubate at 37 °C for 1 h. Add cytokine secretion inhibitors (brefeldin A and monensin) as directed in Table 2 to all wells including the well corresponding to unstimulated control, mix well

by pipetting and continue to incubate the plate at 37 °C, in a CO_2 incubator for an additional 4–5 h (*see* **Note 11**).

(b) Immobilized anti-CD3 + soluble anti-CD28: Coat 10 wells of a U-bottom 96-well plate with 50 μl/well of anti-CD3 (clones OKT3 or UCHT1) as directed in Table 1, and incubate at 37 °C for 2 h or at 4 °C overnight. Use PBS to coat wells corresponding to unstimulated control. Following incubation, wash the wells with RPMI complete using a quick spin (*see* **Note 12**). Transfer 2×10^5 cells/well (in 200 μl of RPMI-ICS) to ten CD3-immobilized wells (making it a total of 2×10^6 cells when pooled). To this, add soluble anti-CD28 as directed in Table 1, and incubate the plate from 24 h to 3 days (*see* **Note 13**) at 37 °C, in a CO_2 humidified incubator. Four hours prior to the end of stimulation, add cytokine secretion inhibitors (brefeldin A and monensin) as directed in Table 2 to all wells including the well corresponding to unstimulated control, and mix well by pipetting.

(c) LPS: To cells in 200 μl/well with 2×10^6 cells in a U-bottom 96-well plate, add LPS as directed in Table 1, and incubate at 37 °C for 6 or 24 h. Four hours prior to the end of stimulation, add cytokine secretion inhibitors (brefeldin A and monensin) as directed in Table 2 to all wells including the well corresponding to unstimulated control, and mix well by pipetting (*see* **Note 14**).

(d) PHA blasts: Set up PHA blasts by transferring 2×10^6 PBMCs/ml to a 75 cm^2 flask (*see* **Note 15**) using RPMI + 20% FBS + Hepes 2 mM + 1% P/S + L-glutamine medium. To this, add PHA-P as directed in Table 1, and place it at 37 °C, in a CO_2 humidified incubator for 1–3 days. Four hours prior to the end of stimulation, add cytokine secretion inhibitors (brefeldin A and monensin) as directed in Table 2 to the flask including cells corresponding to unstimulated control, and mix well by pipetting (*see* **Note 16**).

3. After stimulation, add EDTA to a final concentration of 2 mM, and incubate for 15 min at room temperature (*see* **Note 17**).

4. Transfer the cells into tubes or spin down the plate at $400 \times g$ for 5 min, discard the supernatant, and wash once with 0.2 ml of CyFACS buffer per well (*see* **Note 18**).

3.1.4 Live-Dead Marker Staining

1. Aspirate supernatant and agitate the cell pellet. To each sample, add 0.1 ml of Dota-maleimide Rh103 (5 mg/ml) 1:3000 (or optimal concentration from titration) diluted in PBS, and incubate on ice for 10 min.

2. Wash twice with PBS at 400 × *g* for 5 min.
3. Aspirate supernatant and proceed with barcoding as detailed in the next section.

3.2 Mass Cytometry Staining and Data Acquisition

3.2.1 Barcoding

1. Following aspiration of supernatant, mix the cells with a small volume of PBS left over the top of cell pellet, and transfer cell contents to a 2-ml 96-well deep well plate containing 1 ml of barcode perm buffer (Fluidigm), and wash at 500 × *g* for 5 min.
2. Aspirate and wash again by adding 1 ml of barcode perm buffer per well and centrifuge at 500 × *g* for 5 min (*see* **Note 19**).
3. Resuspend each sample to be barcoded completely in 800 μl of barcode perm buffer (*see* **Note 20**).
4. Resuspend barcodes completely in 100 μl of barcode perm buffer, and transfer them to the appropriate samples. Mix the sample immediately and completely.
5. Incubate for 30 min at room temperature.
6. Following incubation, centrifuge cells at 500 × *g* for 5 min.
7. Discard supernatant, and wash twice with 1 ml of CyFACS buffer per well.
8. Mix cells by adding 0.2 ml of CyFACS buffer per well and pool samples by transferring the cell contents from all wells into a 5-ml Eppendorf Tube corresponding to a sample batch (that will be stained and acquired together on CyTOF) (*see* **Note 21**).

3.2.2 FcR Blocking and Surface Staining

1. Following sample pooling, centrifuge cells at 500 × *g* for 5 min.
2. Aspirate supernatant, and to the pooled pellet, add approximately 150–300 μl (depending on number of samples pooled and pellet size) of FcR blocking solution (Cytodelics) and incubate for 10 min at room temperature (*see* **Note 22**).
3. Without washing off FcR blocking solution, continue with the surface-staining step.
4. Freshly make a mix of surface antibody panel cocktail (*see* Table 3) in CyFACS buffer, and add 150–300 μl (depending on the number of samples pooled and pellet size). For the antibody concentrations, use either Fluidigm-recommended concentration or optimal titer as determined for in-house made conjugates for each antibody.
5. Incubate on ice or in the fridge for 30 min.
6. Wash cells twice using CyFACS buffer at 500 × *g* for 5 min.
7. Discard the supernatant. Dilute 16% (w/v) PFA to 1% (w/v) in PBS, and add 500 μl per sample batch. Fix cells for 10 min at room temperature (if intracellular staining will be performed

Table 3
Surface antibody panel

Metal tag	Marker	Clone	Source
89Y	CD45	HI30	Fluidigm
103Rh	Live–dead	Dota-maleimide	Macrocyclics
115In	CD57	HCD57	BioLegend
142Nd	CD19	HIB19	Fluidigm
143Nd	CD5	UCHT2	BioLegend
144Nd	CD16	3G8	BioLegend
145Nd	CD4	RPA-T4	BioLegend
146Nd	CD8a	SK1	BioLegend
147Sm	CD11c	Bu15	Fluidigm
148Nd	CD31	WM59	BioLegend
154Sm	CD3e	UCHT1	Fluidigm
155Gd	CD7	CD7-6B7	BioLegend
157Gd	CD33	WM53	BioLegend
160Gd	CD14	M5E2	BioLegend
161Dy	CD161	HP-3G10	BioLegend
163Dy	HLA-DR	L243	BioLegend
164Dy	CD44	BJ18	BioLegend
165Ho	CD127	A019D5	Fluidigm
167Er	CD27	L128	Fluidigm
168Er	CD38	HIT2	BioLegend
169Tm	CD45RA	HI100	Fluidigm
170Er	CD20	2H7	BioLegend
172Yb	IgD	IA6-2	BioLegend
173Yb	CD56	NCAM16.2	BD
174Yb	CXCR5	51,505	R&D systems
191/193Ir	DNA Intercalator	–	Fluidigm
209Bi	CD11b	Mac-1	Fluidigm

on the same day) or overnight at 4 °C (if intracellular staining will be done on the following day).

Table 4
Intracellular cytokine staining panel

Metal tag	Marker	Clone	Source
149Sm	IL-4	MP4-25D2	BioLegend
150Nd	IFNγ	B27	BioLegend
153Eu	IL-5	TRFK5	BioLegend
156Gd	IL-6	MQ2-13AS	Fluidigm
158Gd	IL-2	MQ1-17H12	Fluidigm
159 Tb	IL-10	JES3-9D7	BioLegend
166Er	IL-17A	BL168	Biolegend
171Yb	Granzyme B	GB11	Fluidigm
175Lu	TNFα	MAb11	Biolegend

3.2.3 Permeabilization and Intracellular Staining

1. Wash cells twice using CyFACS buffer at 500 × *g* for 5 min.
2. Discard the supernatant, and add *X* μl (calculate 80 μl/sample × number of samples in the pooled batch) of fixation/permeabilization working solution (eBioscience) to each pooled sample pellet and resuspend (*see* **Note 23**).
3. Incubate at room temperature for 30 min.
4. Without washing, add *Y* μl (calculate 170 μl/sample × number of samples in the pooled batch) of 1× permeabilization buffer to each pooled sample pellet and mix.
5. Wash twice at 500 × *g* for 5 min.
6. Discard supernatant and resuspend sample pellet in residual volume with gentle vortexing.
7. Freshly make a mix of intracellular antibody panel cocktail (*see* Table 4) in 1× permeabilization buffer, and add 150–300 μl (depending on number of samples pooled and pellet size). For the antibody concentrations, use either Fluidigm-recommended concentration or optimal titer as determined for in-house made conjugates for each antibody.
8. Incubate for 45 min on ice/in the fridge or 1 h at room temperature.
9. Wash twice with 1× permeabilization buffer at 500 × *g* for 5 min.
10. Aspirate supernatant, and resuspend sample pellet in residual volume with gentle vortexing.
11. Dilute 16% (w/v) PFA to 4% (w/v) in PBS, and add 500 μl per sample batch. Fix cells for 10 min at room temperature

(if fixation was done overnight post surface-staining step) or overnight at 4 °C (if cells were fixed for 10 min post surface-staining step) (*see* **Note 24**).

3.2.4 DNA (Iridium) Staining and Data Acquisition

1. To cells fixed for 10 min/overnight, add DNA iridium intercalator (^{191}Ir/^{193}Ir) diluted 1000× (or optimal concentration from titration) (stock 125 μM) in 4% (w/v) PFA. Add 40 μl (from 1:80 intermediate stock) to 500 μl cell suspension, and incubate for 20 min at room temperature.
2. Wash once in CyFACS buffer (*see* **Note 25**), followed by a wash in PBS 1× at 500 × *g* for 5 min.
3. Proceed to two Milli-Q water washes at 500 × *g* for 5 min.
4. Dilute EQ™ four element calibration beads (Fluidigm) 0.1× in Milli-Q water. These calibration beads allow normalization of data based on standard bead intensities.
5. Count the cells in each sample batch, and adjust the concentration to 7–8 × 10^5 cells/ml using the diluted EQ beads solution.
6. Filter the sample by passing the cell suspension through a strainer cap of a 5-ml tube to remove any cell aggregates that might cause clogging during data acquisition.
7. Acquire data on a CyTOF version 1, CyTOF version 2 or Helios mass cytometer. Acquire the whole sample at 200 to 300 events/s to be able to identify rare cell subsets and low frequencies of cytokine producing cells. *See* Fig. 2 for representative data.

3.3 Example Data Analysis Method

After normalizing and de-barcoding the single-cell data, cell populations typically are defined using traditional manual gating or automated clustering methods [12, 13]. This defines the cell composition of an individual's immune system, a feature recently shown to be stable within an individual over time, but enormously variable between individuals [14].

In each of the identified cell populations, the intracellular markers and functional responses can be further assessed. An example for T cells is shown in Fig. 2a showing variable cytokines and chemokines produced in responses to in vitro PMA/ionomycin stimulation, as a reflection of the functional state of these T cells (Fig. 2a). Interestingly, assessing all 64 possible combinations of these 9 different response mechanisms provides an extraordinarily sensitive measure of immune cell function in various conditions of health and disease. An example is shown in Fig. 2b with the main subpopulations of T cells highlighted, and the many smaller populations combined illustrating the range of variation from 30% to 0% of T cells (Fig. 2b).

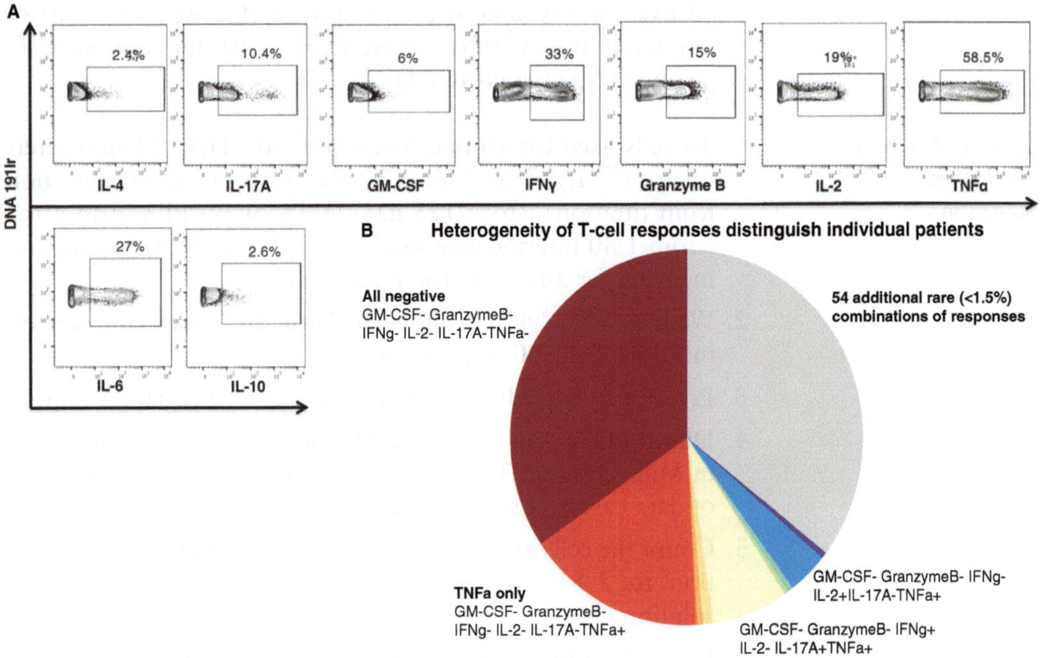

Fig. 2 Representative ICS data obtained from CyTOF. (**a**) Representative data showing individual, intracellular markers induced upon PMA/ionomycin or LPS stimulation. The staining profiles show IL-2, GM-CSF, IFNγ, TNFα secretion by CD3+ T cells and IL-4, IL-5, IL-17A secretion by CD4+ T cells upon PMA/ionomycin stimulation for 5 h; IL-6 and IL-10 secretion by CD14+ monocytes upon LPS stimulation for 5 h. (**b**) A pie chart illustrating the heterogeneity of T cell responses for cytokines based on assessment of 64 possible combinations of response mechanisms

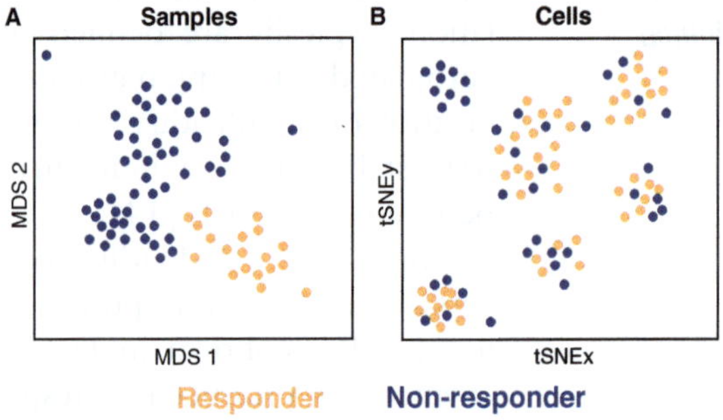

Fig. 3 An illustration showing how more comprehensive measurements can offer greater sensitivity in separating, (**a**) groups of patients by differences in known cell populations, and (**b**) novel cell populations associated with groups of patients

Once these summary statistics are collected, they define the state of an individual's immune system and can be used to compare patients and used as predictors of disease outcome. By comparing samples based on a high number of informative features, the resolution for separating samples based on outcome, such as responsiveness to therapy can likely be increased (Fig. 3a). Such analyses are based on known populations and functional traits, but another informative analysis involves the analysis of single cells and their distribution in different patients, allowing the definition of previously unanticipated cell populations as discriminating features (Fig. 3b). This is a non-exhaustive summary of some of the many possible analyses methods that can be applied in order to understand systems-level features distinguishing patient groups and biological phenomena.

4 Notes

1. CyFACS and PBS 1X buffers should be stored in LDPE (low-density polyethylene) and not glass bottles since glass bottles washed with detergents introduce barium contaminant to the buffers unlike LDPE bottles.
2. Purified antibodies were obtained in carrier/protein-free buffer and then coupled to lanthanide metals using the MaxPar antibody conjugation kit (Fluidigm) [15] as per the protocol obtained from Fluidigm. After determining the protein concentration by measurement of absorbance at 280 nm, the metal-labeled antibodies were diluted in PBS Antibody Stabilization solution (CANDOR Bioscience) for long-term storage at 4 °C. Antibodies used in this study are listed in the Tables 3 and 4.
3. Human PBMCs isolated (using Lymphoprep™-based density gradient centrifugation technique) from whole blood or buffy coats obtained from healthy donors or from whole blood of patients are cryopreserved (using standard PBMC cryopreservation protocol) and thawed for ICS assay.
4. ThawSTAR® offers the advantage in that it has multiple detection systems that determine vial temperature, phase change initiation, and completion of sample thawing. With an automated calibration, ThawSTAR® efficiently determines when a cell is thawed appropriately with minimal cell death during the thaw process.
5. Upon thawing in ThawSTAR® instrument, when the instrument beeps and vial pops out, there could be a part in the vial not completely thawed. The vial can then be vortexed quickly before adding thawing medium and transferring it to a falcon tube containing thawing medium.
6. Thaw a maximum of three samples at a time.

7. RPMI-ICS medium containing 2% FCS is used for ICS assay. Adding more concentration of FBS in this medium will add to unspecific stimulation of cells in addition to the stimulation caused by activating stimuli.
8. Before finalizing study design, test the effect of different resting times for your particular cell type of interest.
9. Human PBMCs isolated (using Lymphoprep^{TM}-based density gradient centrifugation technique) from whole blood or buffy coats obtained from healthy donors or from whole blood of patients freshly used in ICS assay.
10. SepMate tubes (STEMCELL Technologies) offer an advantage in that PBMCs end up above a separation membrane from Lymphoprep^{TM} that minimizes the likelihood of getting Lymphoprep^{TM} into PBMCs as Lymphoprep^{TM} contributes to large amounts of iodine-containing preservatives.
11. Based on the cell sample used, test PMA/ionomycin stimulation from 4–6 h for optimal detection of cytokines secreted.
12. Overnight incubation of the plate at 4 °C with anti-CD3-coated wells offers an efficient co-stimulation of T cells. It is important to wash the coated wells thrice to remove any unbound antibody before addition of cells.
13. Optimal timing conditions for CD3 + CD28 co-stimulation must be tested beforehand using the sample of interest.
14. LPS stimulation conditions vary with the cytokine being tested. For example, 24-h stimulation is needed for detection of IL-10 and MCP-1 secreted by CD14+ monocytes, while 4–6 h is enough to detect IL-1α, IL-1β, IL-6, and IL-8 secreted by CD14+ monocytes.
15. For setting up PHA blasts, the total volume in each flask can be 40–120 ml.
16. Do not use PHA-stimulated donor PBMCs older than 3 days post-stimulation.
17. Pipette cells gently up and down after incubation with EDTA to collect all cells that have adhered to the wells.
18. Collect PHA blasts from culture flask, count, and transfer 2×10^6 cells/sample into a U-bottom 96-well plate for live--dead staining. Similarly, with CD3 + CD28 co-stimulated cells, pool 10 wells/sample with 2×10^5 cells/well and transfer to a U-bottom 96-well plate for live–dead staining.
19. Dilute barcode perm buffer (10×) to 1× using PBS.
20. Each barcode in Fluidigm's Cell-ID 20-Plex Pd Barcoding Kit can be used in a diluted form. Optimal dilution can be tested in your lab based on cell type being used in the assay and the

number of samples that will be barcoded and pooled per each sample batch that will be acquired by CyTOF.

21. Depending on the number of samples barcoded and pooled per batch, transfer the pooled contents into a 5-ml Eppendorf or 15-ml falcon tube and spin down.

22. Optimal amount of antibody cocktail to be added per each pooled batch of barcoded samples should be determined on testing. Roughly, at least around twofold antibody amount can be reduced from what would generally be used if the antibodies were added individually to non-barcoded samples.

23. To samples fixed post surface staining using 1–2% PFA, fix/-perm buffer as a first step (*see* Subheading 3.2.3) in the intracellular staining protocol can be added as this helps in better recovery of cells, following which they are permeabilized using permeabilization buffer (eBioscience).

24. Overnight fixation of cells with PFA at least once either before or after intracellular staining helps in robust fixation of cells that helps in lesser cell loss when samples are washed in Milli-Q water before being acquired by CyTOF.

25. Further to DNA staining and washes in CyFACS buffer, (a) if samples will be acquired during the next 1 or 2 days, they can then be resuspended in CyFACS buffer and left at 4 °C. On the day of acquisition, proceed with PBS and water washes; (b) if samples will be acquired after a week or later, they can be frozen in 150 μl of 10% DMSO/FBS in a U-bottom 96-well plate and stored at −80 °C for 1–3 weeks before acquisition by CyTOF. Cell staining profiles are not compromised upon freezing as compared to refrigeration [16].

References

1. Bandura DR, Baranov VI, Ornatsky OI et al (2009) Mass cytometry: technique for real time single cell multitarget immunoassay based on inductively coupled plasma time-of-flight mass spectrometry. Anal Chem 81:6813–6822
2. Bendall SC, Simonds EF, Qiu P et al (2011) Single-cell mass cytometry of differential immune and drug responses across a human hematopoietic continuum. Science 332:687–696
3. Brodin P, Jojic V, Gao T et al (2015) Variation in the human immune system is largely driven by non-heritable influences. Cell 160:37–47
4. Kaczorowski KJ, Shekhar K, Nkulikiyimfura D et al (2017) Continuous immunotypes describe human immune variation and predict diverse responses. Proc Natl Acad Sci U S A 114:E6097–E6106
5. Wong MT, Ong DE, Lim FS et al (2016) A high-dimensional atlas of human T cell diversity reveals tissue-specific trafficking and cytokine signatures. Immunity 45:442–456
6. Newell EW, Sigal N, Nair N et al (2013) Combinatorial tetramer staining and mass cytometry analysis facilitate T-cell epitope mapping and characterization. Nat Biotechnol 31:623–629
7. Chevrier S, Levine JH, VRT Z et al (2017) An immune atlas of clear cell renal cell carcinoma. Cell 169:736–749 e18
8. Lavin Y, Kobayashi S, Leader A et al (2017) Innate immune landscape in early lung adenocarcinoma by paired single-cell analyses. Cell 169:750–765 e17
9. Lakshmikanth T, Olin A, Chen Y et al (2017) Mass cytometry and topological data analysis

reveal immune parameters associated with complications after allogeneic stem cell transplantation. Cell Rep 20:2238–2250
10. Wei SC, Levine JH, Cogdill AP et al (2017) Distinct cellular mechanisms underlie anti-CTLA-4 and anti-PD-1 checkpoint blockade. Cell 170:1120–1133 e17
11. Phelan MC and Lawler G (2001) Cell counting. Current Protocols in Cytometry 00: A.3A.1–A.3A.4
12. Shekhar K, Brodin P, Davis MM et al (2014) Automatic classification of cellular expression by nonlinear stochastic embedding (ACCENSE). Proc Natl Acad Sci U S A 111:202–207
13. Weber LM, Robinson MD (2016) Comparison of clustering methods for high-dimensional single-cell flow and mass cytometry data. Cytometry A 89:1084–1096
14. Brodin P, Davis MM (2016) Human immune system variation. Nat Rev Immunol 17:21–29
15. Lou X, Zhang G, Herrera I et al (2007) Polymer-based elemental tags for sensitive bioassays. Angew Chem Int Ed 46:6111–6114
16. Sumatoh HR, Teng KW, Cheng Y et al (2017) Optimization of mass cytometry sample cryopreservation after staining. Cytometry A 91:48–61

Chapter 4

Immune Monitoring of Cancer Patients by Multi-color Flow Cytometry

Shi Yong Neo, Aine O'Reilly, and Yago Pico de Coaña

Abstract

The irruption of immune-activating therapies to treat cancer has created a need for evaluating both the response and possible adverse events related to these novel treatments. Multicolor flow cytometry is a powerful tool that enables tumor immunologists to characterize the immune system of patients before and in response to immunotherapy. We present here a protocol for purifying human peripheral blood mononuclear cells and staining them with a set of six multicolor panels that allow for a thorough characterization of the immune system of healthy donors as well as patients that are undergoing treatments that may modify the immune system.

Key words Flow cytometry, Peripheral blood mononuclear cells, Immune monitoring, Immunotherapy, Tumor immunology

1 Introduction

In the last decade, harnessing the power of the immune system has emerged as one of the most promising therapeutic modalities to treat patients with cancer [1]. The oncology field has been revolutionized by two distinct approaches: checkpoint blockade and cellular therapy. The success rates of these therapies, while encouraging, still have a lot of room to increase, with improved survival in 15 to 90% of patients [2–4]. Additionally, immune-related adverse events such as inflammatory intestinal manifestations, hepatitis, and dermatitis can be frequent, especially in the case of checkpoint blockade [5].

There are several translational tools available for monitoring the immune system of patients, and of these, flow cytometry is considered the gold standard due to its versatility, precision, speed, accessibility, and cost-effectiveness [6].

Flow cytometry can be used on any type of source material such as body fluids, blood, tumor, or bone marrow [7]. The limiting factor is that a fluid suspension has to be prepared before analysis.

Yago Pico de Coaña (ed.), *Immune Checkpoint Blockade: Methods and Protocols*, Methods in Molecular Biology, vol. 1913, https://doi.org/10.1007/978-1-4939-8979-9_4, © Springer Science+Business Media, LLC, part of Springer Nature 2019

The characteristics of this technique allow for both phenotypical description and functional assays, providing quantitative and qualitative measurements of distinct parameters. Furthermore, it is regularly applied to assess protein expression, cell viability, and cell enrichment in different clinical preparations.

In this setting, a properly established immune monitoring protocol would allow to take a snapshot of the immune system in patients that are undergoing different treatments, facilitating the search for biomarkers. In parallel, biobanked samples from these patients would be available for functional assays that can allow for a greater understanding of the mechanisms involved in an effective response to treatment, opening the door to the possible improvement of existing therapies and therefore closing the bedside to bench-to-bedside circle.

This chapter contains a detailed protocol that includes all necessary steps to monitor the immune system in patients undergoing different treatments. The six staining panels will allow to determine frequencies of a broad spectrum of cellular populations (Table 1). Panel 1 can determine frequencies of CD4 and CD8 T cells as well as their memory and activation status [8]. Panel number 2 is designed to analyze the regulatory T cell population [9]. Panel number 3 contains a number of functional markers that are present in both T cells and NK cells [8]. The main focus in panel 4 is the NK cell population [10–12]. Panel 5 explores the frequencies of two well characterized myeloid derived suppressor cell (MDSC) populations, of monocytic and polymorphonuclear origin (MoMDSC and PMN-MDSC, respectively) [9, 13, 14]. Panel 6 aims to identify if any of the myeloid populations are positive for the immunosuppressive enzymes Arginase-1 (ARG) and inducible nitric oxide synthase (iNOS) [9].

2 Materials

2.1 Ficoll Density Gradient Centrifugation

1. Polystyrene conical tubes—Falcon (50 ml/15 ml).
2. Serological pipets (5 ml, 10 ml, 25 ml, 50 ml).
3. Ficoll-Paque plus solution (GE Healthcare Bioscience).
4. Phosphate-buffered saline (PBS) pH 7.4: 137 mM NaCl, 2.7 mM KCl, 10 mM $Na_2HPO_4 \cdot \times 2H_2O$, 2 mM KH_2PO_4.
5. Light microscope.
6. Hemocytometer.
7. Refrigerated table top centrifuge with swing bucket rotor and 96-well plate adapter.
8. Freezing medium (90% fetal calf serum, 10% DMSO).

Table 1
Staining panels used for flow cytometry. The volumes (in μl) for each antibody correspond to master mixes calculated for 3.5 stainings

Number	1		2		3		4		5		6	
	T cell memory		**Tregs**		**T cell function**		**NK cells**		**MDSCs**		**Arg/iNOS**	
FITC	CCR5	3.5	**FoxP3**		CD3	7	DNAM-1	14	–	–	–	–
PE	CCR7	7	ICOS	3.5	**TCRζ**		*NKp30/NKp46*	14/3.5	HLA-DR	7	HLA-DR	7
PE-CF594	CD8	7	CD4	7	–	–	–	–	–	–	–	–
PerCP-Cy5.5	CD28	1.75	CD28	1.75	CD4	3.5	HLA-DR	1	CD3/CD19	3.5/7	**iNOS**[a]	
PE-Cy7	CD3	0.9	–	–	CD56	7	CD56	7	CD15	3.5	CD3	0.9
APC	CD45RA	3.5	CD127[a]	17.5	FasL	7	NKG2D	7	CD33	7	CD33	7
APC-Cy7	CD69	1.75	CD8	3.5	CD8	3.5	CD69	1.75	CD11b	3.5	CD11b	3.5
PacBlue	CXCR3	7	CD25	14	PD1	7	CD16	1.75	CD14	1	CD14	1
PacOrange	–	–	–	–	–	–	CD3	14	–	–	**Arg**	
Aqua	DCM		DCM		DCM		–		DCM		–	
DAPI	–		–		–		DCM		–		DCM	
FACS buffer	34.1		22.75		35		6		37.5		50.6	
Notes			**ICS**		**ICS special**						ICS	

[a]CD127 antibody is conjugated with Alf-647

2.2 Flow Cytometry

1. FACS buffer: PBS + human serum albumin to a 1% final concentration. Store at 4 °C.
2. Aqua Dead Cell Marker (Aqua DCM): LIVE/DEAD™ Fixable Aqua Dead Cell Stain Kit, for 405 nm excitation (Thermo Fisher Scientific) (*see* **Note 1**).
3. Ultraviolet Dead Cell Marker (UVDCM): LIVE/DEAD™ Fixable Blue Dead Cell Stain Kit, for UV excitation (Thermo Fisher Scientific) (*see* **Note 1**).
4. IVIg 100 mg ml (Privigen) (*see* **Note 2**).
5. Polypropylene round-bottom tubes (5 ml).
6. 96-well V-bottom plates.
7. Antibodies for flow cytometry (*see* Table 2).
8. Digitonin permeabilizing solution: Digitonin 25 mg/ml in PBS. Dissolve 250 mg digitonin in10 ml PBS in a boiling water bath for 30 min. Let cool to room temperature, and filter first through a 0.80-μm syringe filter and then a through a 0.22-μm syringe filter. After filtering, check if the solution is clear, and discard turbid batches. Prepare 1 ml aliquots and freeze at −20 °C (*see* **Note 3**) [15].
9. Paraformaldehyde (PFA) stock solution: PFA 2% (w/v) in H2O. Add 2 g PFA powder to 100 ml of 1× PBS. Heat to 70 ° C (do not exceed this temperature) in a fume hood until PFA goes into solution. Allow the solution to cool to room temperature. Adjust to pH 7.4 using 0.1 M NaOH or 0.1 M HCl, if needed. Filter and store at 4 ° C protected from light.
10. Fixation/Permeabilization Solution Kit (BD Biosciences).
11. Flow cytometer with at least 11 channels (FSC, SSC + 9) (*see* **Note 4**).
12. Computer with appropriate software for flow cytometry analysis (*see* **Note 5**).
13. Refrigerated benchtop centrifuge with 96-well plate adaptors.

3 Methods

3.1 Initial Considerations for Blood Sampling

The quality of any experiment always begins with sample collection. Thus, it is important to keep high standards of phlebotomy and good biobanking practices. A venipuncture can be routinely performed by a certified healthcare practitioner, but having adequate knowledge of what could compromise the quality of blood collected is useful to rule out potential downstream errors in.

Before any work is started, one should consider if the anticoagulant used during sample collection is suitable for the study. In recent years, many studies involve assessing metabolism of PBMCs

Table 2
Antibodies used for staining

Marker	Fluorochrome	Clone	Supplier
Arg	PO[a]	6G3	Hycult Biotech
CCR5	FITC	HEK/1/85a	BioLegend
CCR7	PE	150,503	BD Biosciences
CD3	FITC	UCHT1	BD Biosciences
CD3	PerCP-Cy5.5	SK7	BioLegend
CD3	PE-Cy7	UCHT1	BioLegend
CD3	PO	UCHT1	Invitrogen
CD4	PE-CF594	RPA-T4	BD Biosciences
CD4	PerCp-Cy5.5	SK3	BioLegend
CD8	APC-Cy7	SK1	BioLegend
CD11b	APC-Cy7	ICRF44	BD Biosciences
CD14	PB	M5E2	BioLegend
CD15	PE-Cy7	HI98	BD Biosciences
CD16	PB	3G8	BD Biosciences
CD19	PerCP-Cy5.5	HIB19	BD Biosciences
CD25	PB	BC96	BioLegend
CD28	PerCP-Cy5.5	CD28.2	BioLegend
CD33	APC	WM53	BioLegend
CD45RA	APC	HI100	BioLegend
CD56	PE-Cy7	HCD56	BioLegend
CD69	APC-Cy7	FN50	BioLegend
CD127	Alf647	A019D5	BioLegend
CXCR3	PB	G025H7	BioLegend
DNAM-1	FITC	DX11	BD Biosciences
FasL	APC	NOK-1	Miltenyi Biotec
FoxP3	FITC	PCH101	eBioscience
HLA-DR	PE	L243	BioLegend
HLA-DR	PerCP-Cy5.5	G46-6	BD Biosciences
ICOS	PE	DX29	BD Biosciences
iNOS	PerCP	PC	Santa Cruz Biotech
NKG2D	APC	1D11	BioLegend

(continued)

Table 2
(continued)

Marker	Fluorochrome	Clone	Supplier
NKp30	PE	Z256	Beckman Coulter
NKp46	PE	BAB281	Beckman Coulter
PD1	PB	EH12.2H7	BioLegend
TCRZeta	PE	2H2D9	Beckman Coulter

[a]Conjugated with Zenon® Pacific Orange™ Mouse IgG_1 Labeling Kit (Invitrogen)

or purified immune cell subsets [16–19]. The anticoagulant of choice could potentially alter metabolism of the cells before we even start any in vitro assays. For instance, EDTA, while being the anticoagulatory of choice for nucleic acid purification, is a chelator of calcium ions and might affect the study of membrane ion flux and mitochondria. Heparin (lithium or potassium), on the other hand, is the routine anticoagulant of choice used for studying immune populations.

Despite having skilled and knowledgeable phlebotomists, one should still anticipate blood samples that might not be in the desired conditions. Often clinicians encounter frail patients with less visible veins and would possibly apply the tourniquet for too long, causing some cell lysis in the blood collected. In this situation, a decision should be made whether proceeding with the experiment is possible. However, careful consideration should be exercised before discarding any clinical samples especially if they are part of a longitudinal immune monitoring study.

3.2 Isolation of Peripheral Blood Mononuclear Cells

1. Distribute blood into 50-ml Falcon tubes (12–18 ml/tube).
2. Add sterile PBS to a final 35-ml volume in each Falcon. Mix by pipetting up and down.
3. Deposit 10 ml of Ficoll in a fresh 50-ml tube.
4. Carefully overlay the PBS-blood mixture on top of the Ficoll (*see* **Note 6**).
5. Centrifuge for 22 min at 800 × *g* with acceleration and break turned off.
6. After centrifugation is done, gently move the tubes to a laminar flow hood and check for red blood cell lysis (*see* **Notes 7** and **8**).
7. Draw off the upper layer using a pipette, leaving the lymphocyte layer undisturbed at the interface (*see* **Note 9**). The upper layer of plasma may be saved for later use.
8. Using a 5-ml pipette, transfer the lymphocyte layer to a 50-ml Falcon tube. Pool two Ficoll layers per tube. It is critical to

remove all of the interface but a minimum amount of Ficoll and supernatant. Removing excess Ficoll causes granulocyte contamination; removing excess supernatant results in unnecessary contamination by platelets and plasma proteins.

9. Add sterile PBS to a final volume of 50 ml.
10. Centrifuge at 450 × *g* for 7 min.
11. Discard supernatant, resuspend pellet, pool all the tubes, and resuspend in 35-ml sterile PBS (*see* **Note 10**).
12. Centrifuge at 300 × *g* for 7 min.
13. Repeat **steps 9** and **10**.
14. Resuspend in 2.75-ml PBS and count cells.

3.3 Defining Flow Cytometer Application Settings and Compensation for a Prospective Study

Quality control of the machine used during the immune monitoring of patient samples is essential. In our facility, day-to-day variations are measured using cytometer setup and tracking (CS&T) beads. In addition to that, we follow strict application setup for our flow cytometer in order to ensure consistency of results over time as recommended in by BD biosciences [20].

Regarding compensation, if application settings are properly and efficiently characterized in the flow cytometer, it should only be calculated at the beginning of the study, and each time a new lot of any of the antibodies is used to replace a spent reagent (*see* **Note 11**).

3.4 Staining for Flow Cytometry

During the staining procedure, all incubations take place in the dark at 4 °C unless stated otherwise.

1. Prepare antibody master mixes according to Table 2 (*see* **Note 12**).
2. Add 3 × 10^5 cells/well to a 96-well V-bottom plate. Add 100 μl PBS to each well, and spin 3 min at 700 × *g*. Prepare the unstained control by adding 5 × 10^5 cells to a 5-ml polypropylene round-bottom tube and 500 μl FACS buffer.
3. Prepare DCM: 1 μl stock + 1000 μl PBS. Add 200 μl/sample. Panels 1, 2, 3, and 5 are stained with Aqua DCM. Panels 4 and 6 DCM (Table 2). Incubate 10–15 min at 4 °C protected from light (*see* **Note 13**).
4. Add 200 μl FACS buffer, centrifuge 3 min at 700 × *g*, 4 °C. Repeat wash step (*see* **Notes 14** and **15**).
5. Discard supernatant, add 1 μl IVIg/well, resuspend, and incubate for 5 min at 4 °C in the dark (*see* **Note 13**).
6. Add the appropriate master mix to each well for extracellular staining. Incubate for 20–30 min at 4 °C in the dark.
7. While staining, centrifuge the leftover PBMCs for 5 min, 400 × *g*. Resuspend in freezing medium at 20 × 10^6 cells/ml, and aliquot according to future use (*see* **Note 16**).

8. After extracellular staining is complete, add 200 μl FACS buffer to each well and centrifuge 3 min at 700 × *g*, 4 °C. Repeat wash step.
9. Add 200 μl FACS buffer to the wells with only extracellular staining panels (1, 4, and 5), and transfer from the plate to 5-ml polypropylene round-bottom tubes. Keep tubes at 4 °C in the dark until acquired with the flow cytometer.
10. Start permeabilization for wells 2 and 6: add 100 μl Fixation/Permeabilization Solution Kit, and incubate 15–20 min at 4 °C (*see* **Note 17**).
11. During incubation begin preparing the Arginase-PO conjugated antibody. In a brown Eppendorf Tube labeled as "Arg Ab mix," add 2 μl Arg antibody + 1 μl Zenon Pacific Orange labeling reagent. Incubate for 5 min at RT. Add 1 μl blocking reagent and incubate for another 5 min at RT.
12. To the "Arg Ab" mix Eppendorf, add 14 μl BD Perm/Wash buffer + 2 μl iNOS antibody for a final volume of 20 μl "Arg Ab" mix.
13. After the permeabilization incubation time has ended, wash the plate twice with 200 μl BD Perm/Wash buffer (centrifuge at 700 × *g*, 3 min, 4 °C).
14. After washing, add 4 μl FoxP3 antibody and 16 μl BD Perm/Wash buffer to well 2.
15. Add 19.5 μl of the "Arg Ab," mix to well 6, and incubate 40 min at 4 °C in the dark.
16. Wash twice with 200 μl BD Perm/Wash buffer (700 × *g*, 3 min, 4 °C).
17. Resuspend in 200 μl FACS buffer and transfer samples to FACS tubes. Keep tubes at 4 °C in the dark until acquired with the flow cytometer.
18. Add 100 μl 0.25% PFA to well 3 and transfer its contents to a new plate: incubate for 10 min at room temperature (*see* **Note 18**).
19. Add 100 μl FACS buffer centrifuge 3 min at 700 × *g*, 4 °C. Repeat wash step.
20. Add 94 μl FACS buffer + 1 μl digitonin permeabilizing solution, 5 μl TCR-ζ antibody; incubate 40 min at RT.
21. Add 100 μl FACS buffer centrifuge 3 min at 700 × *g*, 4 °C. Repeat wash step.
22. Resuspend in 200 μl FACS buffer and transfer 5-ml polypropylene round-bottom tubes. Keep tubes at 4 °C in the dark until acquired with the flow cytometer.
23. Acquire samples in the flow cytometer (*see* **Note 19**).

3.5 Data Analysis

After exporting the data from the flow cytometer, an initial gating should be applied to all samples (Fig. 1). In this gating, debris, dead cells, and doublets will be excluded, and all subsequent analysis will be performed on live, single PBMCs.

Subsequent gating strategies for the determination of cellular populations can be seen in Figs. 2, 3, 4, 5, 6, and 7.

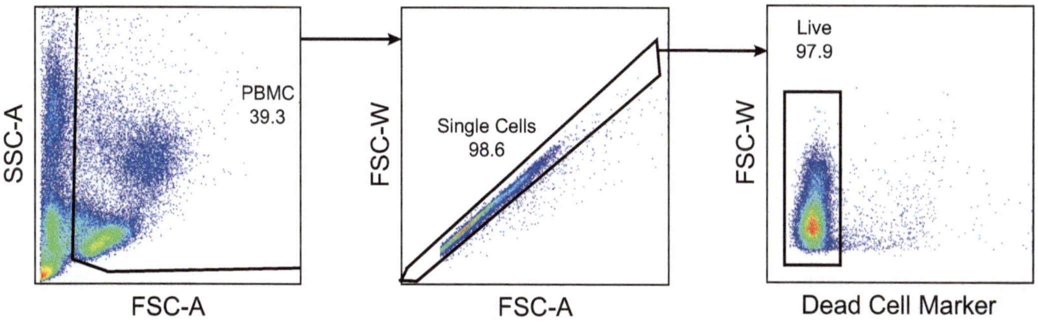

Fig. 1 Singlets and live cells gating strategy (*see* **Notes 20** and **21**)

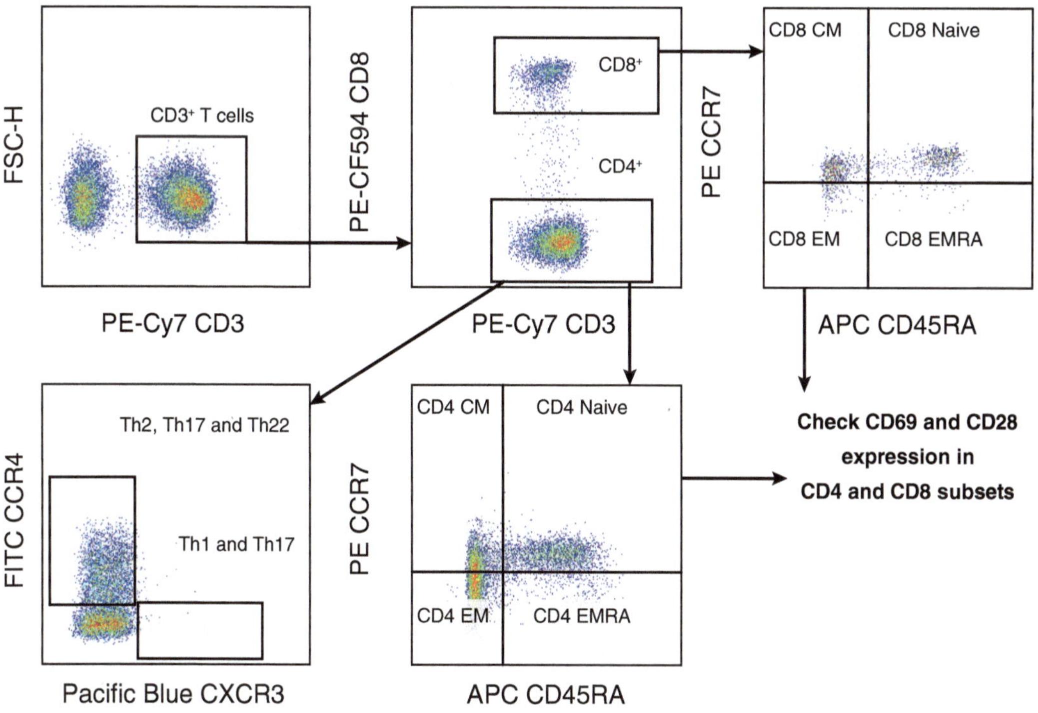

Fig. 2 Gating strategy for panel 1. Using CCR7 and CD45RA, CD4, and CD8 T cells can be subdivided into four major stages of differentiation phenotypes (*see* **Note 22**): CM, Central Memory; EM, Effector memory; EMRA, Effector memory reactivated. Additionally, CD4 T cells can be further subclassified into different Th subpopulations using this panel. CD69 and CD28 can also be used to check the activation status in any of the defined subpopulations

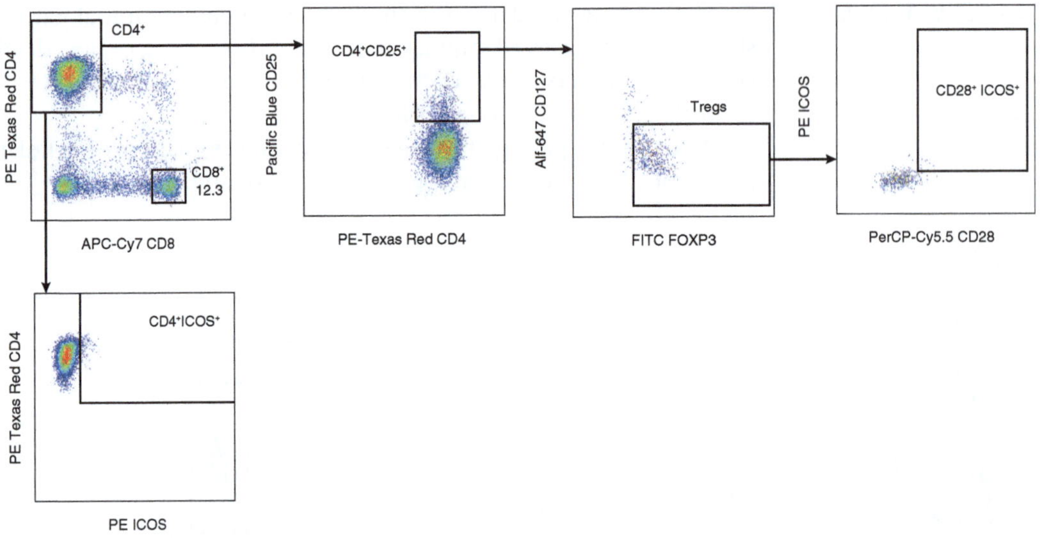

Fig. 3 Gating strategy for panel 2. The main objective of this panel is to quantify Tregs which are defined as $CD4^{+}CD25^{+}CD127^{low}FoxP3^{+}$. ICOS is another T cell activation marker activation marker. It can be measured in the total CD4 or CD 8 T cell populations or in Tregs (*see* **Notes 22** and **23**)

4 Notes

1. We dissolve the original reagent in 50 μl of the provided DMSO and then make 1 μl aliquots in brown Eppendorf tubes, which can be used directly for compensation or frozen and diluted 1:1000 in PBS to stain samples when needed.
2. We use IVIg as an Fc receptor blocking reagent. Other blocking reagents work equally well.
3. Digitonin is toxic in contact with the skin and can be fatal if inhaled. Please use appropriate protective gloves, clothing, and eye and respiratory protection when handling.
4. We use a BD LSRII with the configuration shown in Table 3.
5. We currently use FlowJo v10 (FlowJo, LLC, USA).
6. We use an unorthodox procedure in our lab. Instead of overlaying the PBS-blood mixture on top of the Ficoll, we underlay the Ficoll beneath the blood mixture. To do this, take up 13-ml Ficoll-Paque with a 10-ml pipette, and put it into a 50-ml falcon with the PBS-blood mixture. Make sure that the pipette tip is at the bottom of the tube. Detach the Pipetboy from the Falcon, and let the Ficoll solution flow under the PBS/blood layer by gravity. When the Ficoll has stopped flowing, use your index finger to plug the end of the pipette and carefully remove it. Deposit only 10 ml of Ficoll in the tube and discard the rest.

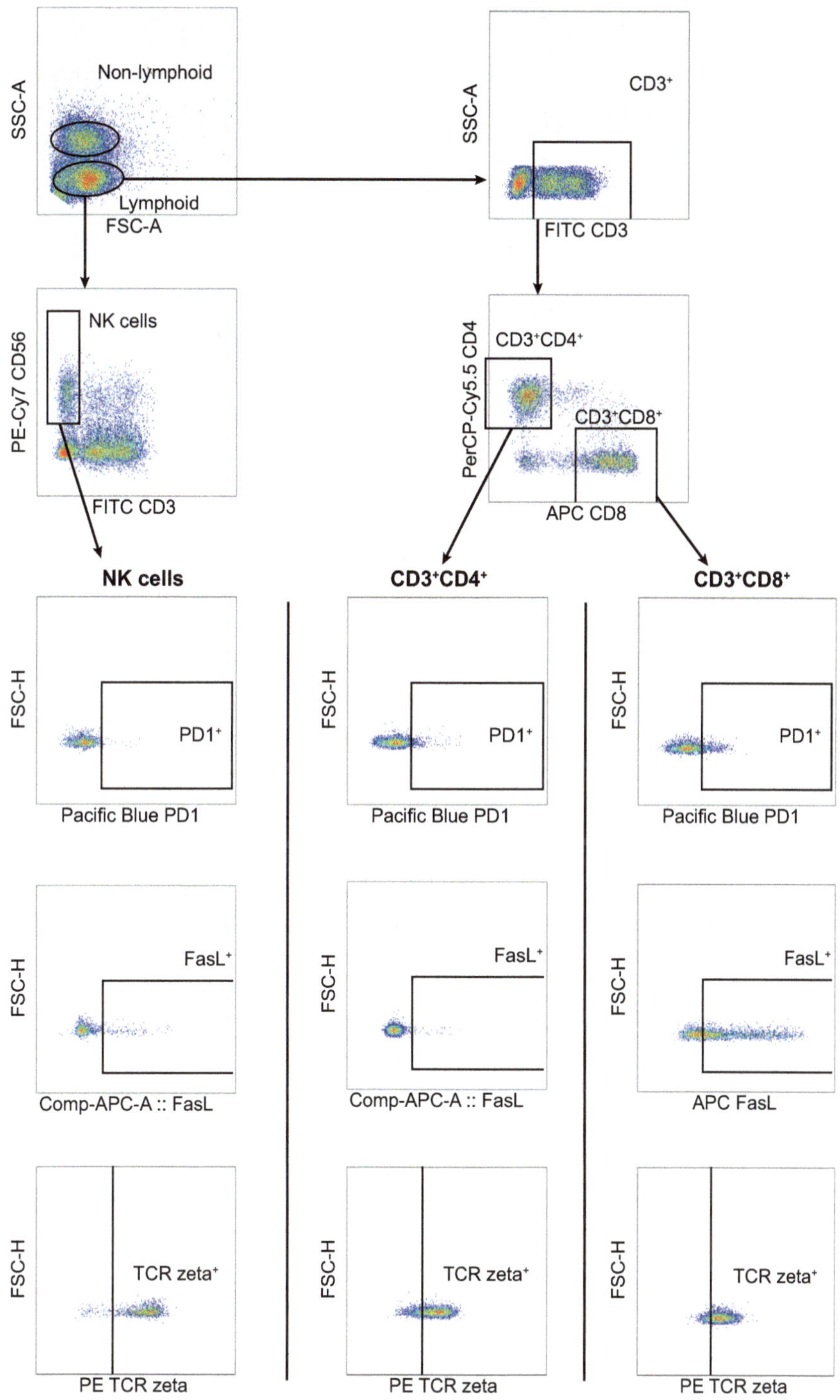

Fig. 4 Gating strategy for panel 3, which is focused on functional markers of T and NK cells. The first step in analyzing this panel is to establish the target populations. On one hand, CD4 and CD8 T cells and on the other hand, NK cells (which are defined as $CD3^{-}CD56^{+}$ lymphoid cells). In these cells, expression levels of functional proteins critical for responses such as Fas-L and TCR-ζ in addition to the immune checkpoint PD-1are reflective of the responses of T and NK cells (*see* **Notes 24–26**)

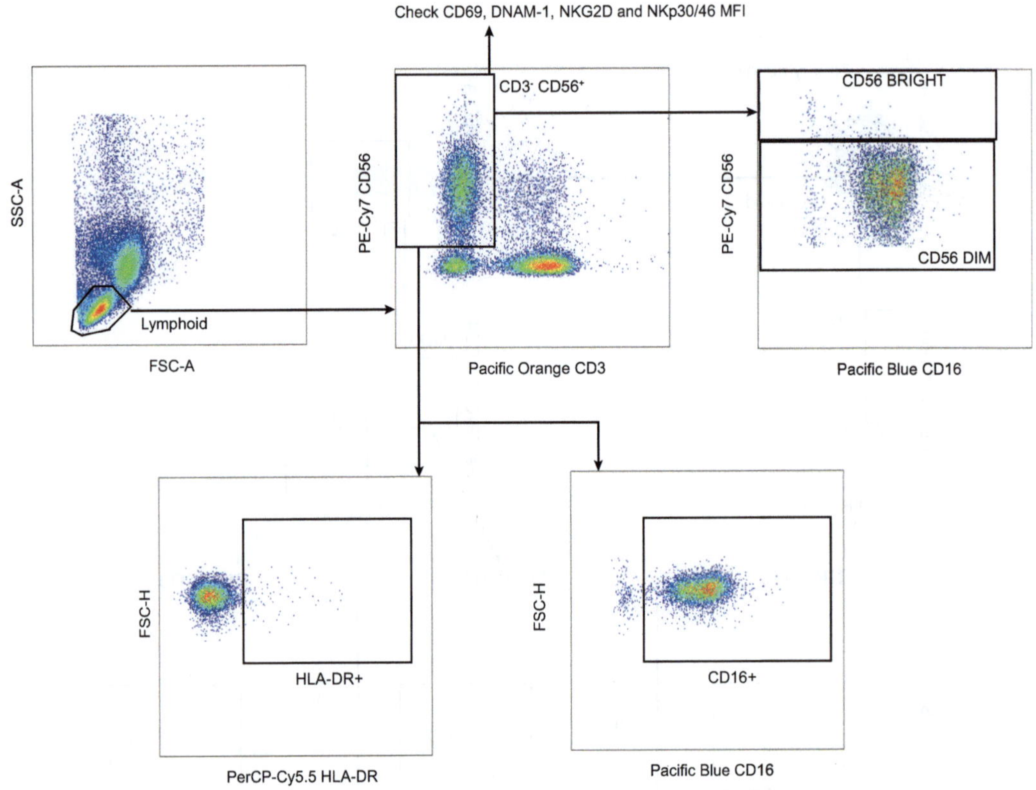

Fig. 5 Gating strategy for panel 4. On the lymphocyte population, NK cells are defined as CD3 negative and CD56 positive. The CD3$^-$CD56+ population are further evaluated using CD56 and CD16 and divided into CD56dim and CD56bright populations. Each resultant subset can then be analyzed for markers of activation such as CD69, expression of activation receptors NKG2D, DNAM-1, and NKp30 combined with NKp46 and markers of functional status such as HLA-DR

7. To detect cell lysis, observe the buffy coat and the plasma fraction of the blood sample for a red coloration after centrifugation. Having cell lysis in our PBMC may or may not affect the outcome of our experiment, but it is a good practice to take note of such observation.
8. Extra care should be taken when moving tubes after gradient separation. Sudden movements can disturb the layers and result in mixing.
9. Although care not to disturb the lymphocyte layer should be taken, be generous while drawing off the upper layer. The more removed the easier the lymphocyte layer will be to visualize.
10. Gently discard the supernatant in a single swift motion. Shaking the tube can cause the pellet to become dislodged.
11. When carrying out a longitudinal study, it is convenient to estimate the total amount of antibodies needed and contact

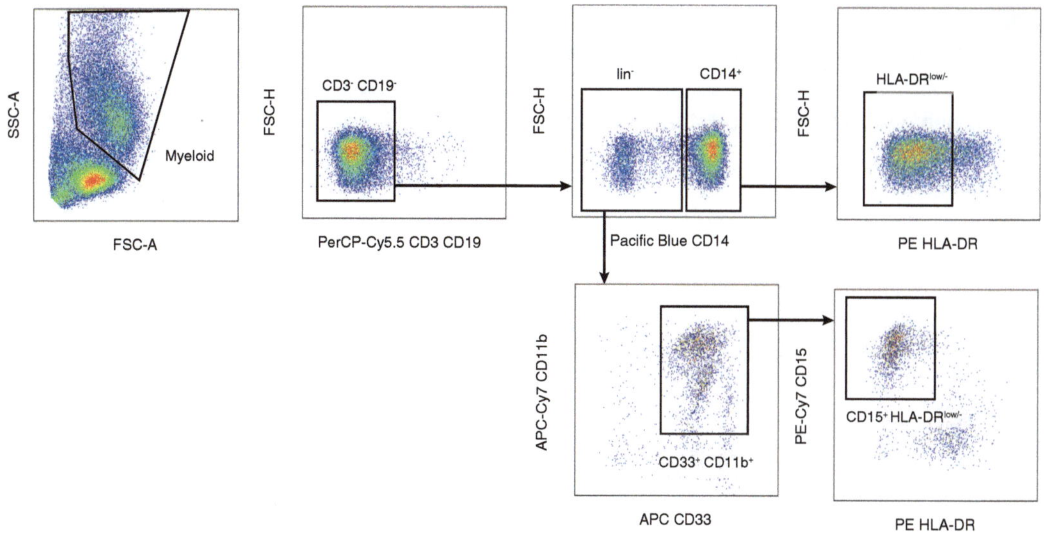

Fig. 6 Gating strategy for panel 5. This panel is focused on determining frequencies of myeloid populations. The first step is to exclude lymphoid cells from the myeloid population by FSC and SSC gating (*see* **Note 27**). The myeloid population is further defined as being negative for CD19 and CD3. Monocytic MDSCs (MoMDSCs) are defined as CD14$^-$ HLA-DR$^{low/-}$. Polymorphonuclear MDSCs (PMN-MDSCs) gating starts from lineage negative cells (lin$^-$):CD3$^-$ CD19$^-$ CD14$^-$; the lin$^-$ population is then gated as CD33$^+$ CD11b$^+$ CD15$^+$ HLA-DR$^{low/-}$ to define PMN-MDSC (*see* **Note 28**)

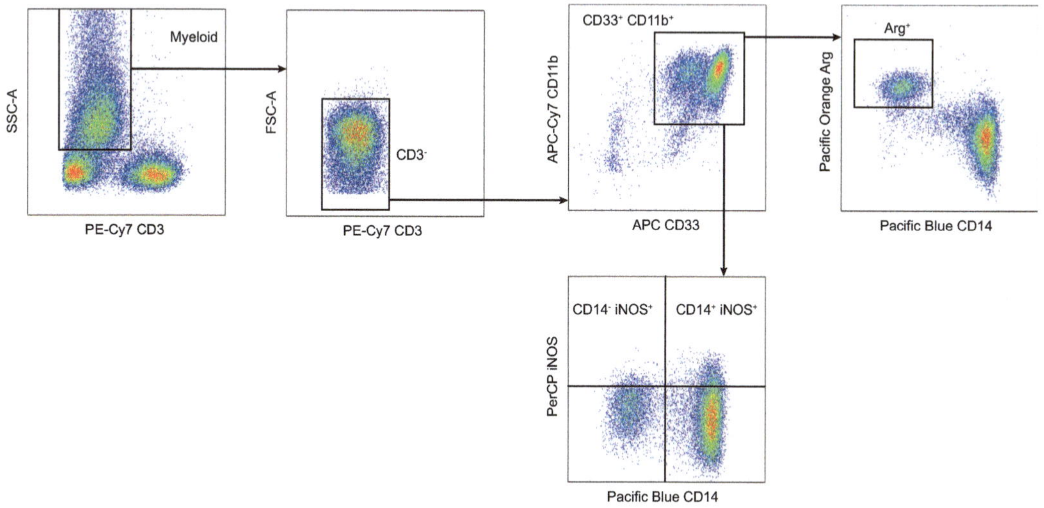

Fig. 7 Gating strategy for panel 6. This panel measures ARG and iNOS in monocytic (CD14$^+$) and PMN (CD14$^-$) myeloid cells (*see* **Note 29**)

suppliers in order to try and purchase large amounts of antibodies with the same lot number.

12. The amounts in the table correspond to the volume of each antibody (in μl) needed to prepare enough master mix to stain

Table 3
BD Biosciences LSRII flow cytometer configuration

Laser name	Wavelength	Detector array	Detector	Channel	Mirror	Filter	Parameter
Blue	488	Octagon	A	5	735 LP	780/60 BP	PE-Cy7
			B	4	680 LP	712/21 BP	PerCP-Cy5-5
			C	3	635 LP	670/14 BP	PerCP
			D	2	595 LP	610/20 BP	PE-CF594
			E	13	555 LP	575/26 BP	PE
			F	12	505 LP	530/30 BP	FITC
			G	1		488/10 BP	SSC
Violet	407	Trigon	A	7	555 LP	585/42 BP	Pacific Orange
			B	6	505 LP	525/50 BP	Aqua DCM
			C	14		450/50 BP	Pacific Blue
325 UV	325	Trigon	B	8	505 LP	450/50 BP	DAPI
Red	633	Trigon	A	11	735 LP	780/60 BP	APC-Cy7
			C	15		660/20 BP	APC
							Alexa Fluor 647

3.5 samples with each antibody. The extra amount is used to take into account possible losses. Master mixes can be stored for up to 3 weeks in brown Eppendorf tubes at 4 °C. Antibody manufacturers recommend giving the mixes a short pulse in a microfuge prior to use, in order to discard aggregates.

13. During staining, it is essential to protect fluorescent reagents and conjugated antibodies from light. We recommend turning off the lights in the flow hood. Additionally, tandem conjugated antibodies are sensitive to temperature. The ideal setting for undisturbed incubations in the dark and at 4 °C is a lidded styrofoam box half full with ice.
14. Discard supernatant in a single swift motion. Repeatedly tipping the plate will result in pellets becoming dislodged.
15. Each time the supernatant is discarded check that a pellet is still present in each well.
16. Deciding the number of cells each aliquot will have depends largely on future downstream applications and biobanking permits. A good starting point is to freeze small (5 million cells/tube) and large (20 million cells/tube) batches. In any case, cryovials should be counted and labeled prior to adding the freezing medium to the cells, to reduce their exposure to DMSO before freezing.

17. **Steps 10–17** apply to permeabilization and staining of wells 2 and 6. **Steps 18–22** correspond to the special permeabilization with digitonin for the TCR-ζ staining. They can be done simultaneously by an experienced researcher, provided that tubes are properly labeled beforehand and multiple lab timers are used.
18. The nature of the TCR-ζ receptor requires a special permeabilization protocol using digitonin.
19. Briefly vortex each sample immediately before acquisition. If the samples have been sitting for a while, the cells will gather at the bottom of the tube.
20. Single cells gating can also be done by plotting SSC area against SSC height or width.
21. Live cells could be present in more than 1 population if cells are permeabilized or have been stimulated with PMA/ionomycin.
22. CCR7 could be replaced by CD27 for the similar gating. CD45RO is a good control, whereby cells positive for CD45RA will be negative for CD45RO. Adding CD27 and CD45RO on top of the panel might be particularly useful to gate the right subsets if the separation of the 4 subsets in the cell plot is unclear with CCR7 against CD45RA.
23. Most regulatory T cells should be low or negative for CD127 unless stimulated.
24. FOXP3 could be upregulated due to T cell stimulation as well. We should hence be cautious and have more stringent gating on only those cells that are highly positive for CD25 and FOXP3.
25. Unlike the PD-1 and FasL, we should use histogram to check the expression levels of TCR zeta assuming all T cells and NK cells should be positive for TCR zeta.
26. Most of the time, healthy and unstimulated PBMC samples show negative PD-1 staining. We could either design a stimulation assay to test for its upregulation as a response by the cells. Apart from that, it is noteworthy that immune checkpoints like PD-1 can be transiently expressed.
27. The lymphoid population can be used as a negative control for all the myeloid markers as they should mostly be negative. This is useful when we are unsure how to define positive populations within the myeloid cell plots.
28. In the gating of CD11b against CD33, it can be common to observe four populations of $CD33^{+}$ $CD11b^{+}$ cells. This is mainly due to different expression levels of the myeloid marker CD33.
29. Expression of ARG and iNOS should be negative in lymphocytes. Gating CD3 positive cells should serve as a negative control.

References

1. Whiteside TL, Demaria S, Rodriguez-Ruiz ME, Zarour HM, Melero I (2016) Emerging opportunities and challenges in cancer immunotherapy. Clin Cancer Res 22(8):1845–1855. https://doi.org/10.1158/1078-0432.CCR-16-0049
2. Lim WA, June CH (2017) The principles of engineering immune cells to treat cancer. Cell 168(4):724–740. https://doi.org/10.1016/j.cell.2017.01.016
3. Pico de Coana Y, Choudhury A, Kiessling R (2015) Checkpoint blockade for cancer therapy: revitalizing a suppressed immune system. Trends Mol Med 21(8):482–491. https://doi.org/10.1016/j.molmed.2015.05.005
4. Weiden J, Tel J, Figdor CG (2018) Synthetic immune niches for cancer immunotherapy. Nat Rev Immunol 18(3):212–219. https://doi.org/10.1038/nri.2017.89
5. Michot JM, Bigenwald C, Champiat S, Collins M, Carbonnel F, Postel-Vinay S et al (2016) Immune-related adverse events with immune checkpoint blockade: a comprehensive review. Eur J Cancer 54:139–148. https://doi.org/10.1016/j.ejca.2015.11.016
6. Finak G, Langweiler M, Jaimes M, Malek M, Taghiyar J, Korin Y et al (2016) Standardizing flow Cytometry Immunophenotyping analysis from the human immunophenotyping consortium. Sci Rep 6:20686. https://doi.org/10.1038/srep20686
7. Adan A, Alizada G, Kiraz Y, Baran Y, Nalbant A (2017) Flow cytometry: basic principles and applications. Crit Rev Biotechnol 37 (2):163–176. https://doi.org/10.3109/07388551.2015.1128876
8. Poschke I, De Boniface J, Mao Y, Kiessling R (2012) Tumor-induced changes in the phenotype of blood-derived and tumor-associated T cells of early stage breast cancer patients. Int J Cancer 131(7):1611–1620. https://doi.org/10.1002/ijc.27410
9. Pico de Coana Y, Poschke I, Gentilcore G, Mao Y, Nystrom M, Hansson J et al (2013) Ipilimumab treatment results in an early decrease in the frequency of circulating granulocytic myeloid-derived suppressor cells as well as their Arginase1 production. Cancer Immunol Res 1(3):158–162. https://doi.org/10.1158/2326-6066.CIR-13-0016
10. Veluchamy JP, Delso-Vallejo M, Kok N, Bohme F, Seggewiss-Bernhardt R, van der Vliet HJ et al (2017) Standardized and flexible eight colour flow cytometry panels harmonized between different laboratories to study human NK cell phenotype and function. Sci Rep 7:43873. https://doi.org/10.1038/srep43873
11. Elisa M, Del ZG, Della CM, Cristina MM, Alessandro M, De MA et al (2013) Human NK cell receptors/markers: a tool to analyze NK cell development, subsets and function. Cytometry A 83(8):702–713. https://doi.org/10.1002/cyto.a.22302
12. Erick TK, Brossay L (2016) Phenotype and functions of conventional and non-conventional NK cells. Curr Opin Immunol 38:67–74. https://doi.org/10.1016/j.coi.2015.11.007
13. Poschke I, Kiessling R (2012) On the armament and appearances of human myeloid-derived suppressor cells. Clin Immunol 144 (3):250–268. https://doi.org/10.1016/j.clim.2012.06.003
14. Pico de Coana Y, Wolodarski M, Poschke I, Yoshimoto Y, Yang Y, Nystrom M et al (2017) Ipilimumab treatment decreases monocytic MDSCs and increases CD8 effector memory T cells in long-term survivors with advanced melanoma. Oncotarget 8 (13):21539–21553. https://doi.org/10.18632/oncotarget.15368
15. Lazarus AH, Ellis J, Blanchette V, Freedman J, Sheng-Tanner X (1998) Permeabilization and fixation conditions for intracellular flow cytometric detection of the T-cell receptor zeta chain and other intracellular proteins in lymphocyte subpopulations. Cytometry 32 (3):206–213
16. Yang R, Lirussi D, Thornton TM, Jelley-Gibbs DM, Diehl SA, Case LK et al (2015) Mitochondrial Ca(2+) and membrane potential, an alternative pathway for interleukin 6 to regulate CD4 cell effector function. Elife 4:e06376. https://doi.org/10.7554/eLife.06376
17. MacIver NJ, Michalek RD, Rathmell JC (2013) Metabolic regulation of T lymphocytes. Annu Rev Immunol 31:259–283. https://doi.org/10.1146/annurev-immunol-032712-095956
18. Palmer CS, Duette GA, Wagner MCE, Henstridge DC, Saleh S, Pereira C et al (2017) Metabolically active CD4+ T cells expressing Glut1 and OX40 preferentially harbor HIV during in vitro infection. FEBS Lett 591 (20):3319–3332. https://doi.org/10.1002/1873-3468.12843
19. Schurich A, Pallett Laura J, Jajbhay D, Wijngaarden J, Otano I, Gill Upkar S et al (2016) Distinct metabolic requirements of

exhausted and functional virus-specific CD8 T cells in the same host. Cell Rep 16 (5):1243–1252. https://doi.org/10.1016/j.celrep.2016.06.078

20. Meinelt E, Reunanen M, Edinger M, Jaimes M, Stall A, Sasaki D et al. (2012) Standardizing application setup across multiple flow cytometers using BD FACSDiva™ Version 6 Software. Technical document. BD biosciences. http://www.bdbiosciences.com/documents/BD_FACSDiva_Stndrd_App_Setup_TechBulletin.pdf

[illegible]

Chapter 5

High-Throughput, Fast, and Sensitive Immunopeptidomics Sample Processing for Mass Spectrometry

Fabio Marino, Chloe Chong, Justine Michaux, and Michal Bassani-Sternberg

Abstract

Comprehensive knowledge of the HLA class I and class II peptides presented to T cells is crucial for designing innovative therapeutics against cancer and other diseases. So far, methodologies for recovery of HLA class I and II peptides for subsequent mass spectrometry-based analysis have been a major limitation. In this chapter we describe a detailed protocol for a high-throughput, reproducible, and sensitive immunoaffinity-purification of HLA-I and HLA-II peptides from up to 96 samples in a plate format, suitable for tissue samples and cell lines. Our methodology reduces sample handling, has a competitive peptide yield, and can be completed within 5 h. This simplified pipeline is applicable for basic and clinical applications.

Key words Immunopeptidomics, Human leukocyte antigen, Antigen processing and presentation, Affinity purification, Mass spectrometry, HLA class I and HLA class II

1 Introduction

The human leukocyte antigen class I (HLA-I) and class II (HLA-II) complexes present to the immune system a highly rich repertoire of peptides (HLAp) derived from degradation of endogenous and exogenous proteins [1]. Antigen processing and presentation is a dynamic process, and the repertoire of the presented immunopeptidome is constantly being shaped by protein expression levels, posttranslational modifications, and the activity of the cellular antigen processing and presentation machinery. Thus, profound alterations on the presented peptidome can arise due to cellular perturbation at multiple levels [2]. HLAp may be derived from disease-related antigens. Therefore, the comprehensive knowledge of the HLAp presented to T cells is crucial for designing innovative therapeutics against cancer, autoimmunity, and pathogenic infections. Presently, mass spectrometry (MS) is the only methodology enabling in-depth characterization of the HLAp in human cell lines

Yago Pico de Coaña (ed.), *Immune Checkpoint Blockade: Methods and Protocols*, Methods in Molecular Biology, vol. 1913, https://doi.org/10.1007/978-1-4939-8979-9_5, © Springer Science+Business Media, LLC, part of Springer Nature 2019

[3–5], tumor tissues [6–8], and body fluids such as plasma [9]. Pioneering studies have already demonstrated that MS-based immunopeptidomics has matured to the extent that the direct identification of clinically relevant neo-antigens has become achievable, which could be exploited for the design of personalized cancer vaccines [10–13]. However, this methodology is still deemed as difficult to implement with low throughput and sensitivity; therefore, it is not ready yet for implementation in clinical settings [14].

MS-based immunopeptidomics workflow involves three main steps: (1) immunoaffinity purification (IP) of HLA complexes followed by extraction and purification of the HLAp, (2) separation of the peptides by chromatography and injection into a MS instrument, and (3) identification of the peptides using search engine tools and bioinformatics. With such a workflow and the new generations of MS, it has become feasible to robustly identify thousands of HLAp per biological sample [5, 15]. One of the bottlenecks of the immunopeptidomics pipeline is the sample preparation procedure, as this determines the overall peptide yield and reproducibility. Usually, this step is time-consuming (3–5 days) and of low throughput [16]. The abovementioned obstacles have led to the slow implementation of this method in the clinic [17]. In this book chapter, we describe a detailed protocol enabling high-throughput extraction of HLAp for MS-based immunopeptidomics [2]. The protocol is applicable for tissue samples and for cell lines. We will focus here on the processing of tissue samples as these are more difficult to handle. We envision that our pipeline will accelerate the development of personalized cancer vaccines and assist in its implementation in clinical practices.

2 Materials

Prepare all solutions with ultrapure water and analytical grade reagents. It is advisable to rinse bottles before use and to employ freshly prepare solutions.

2.1 Purification of Anti-Pan HLA Antibodies from Hybridoma Growth Medium

1. 5 mL of growth medium from HB95 hybridoma cells (ATCC® HB-95™) secreting the W6-32 anti-pan HLA-I and from HB145 hybridoma cells (ATCC® HB-145™) secreting the IVA12 anti pan-HLA-II (*see* **Note 1**).
2. 1% SDS.
3. Ultrapure water.
4. Beads: Protein A-Sepharose® 4B Conjugate.
5. Bio-Spin® disposable chromatography columns (Bio-Rad) with a stand.
6. 100 mM Tris–HCl pH 8.
7. 20 mM Tris–HCl pH 8.

8. 0.1 N acetic acid pH 3.
9. 1 M Tris–HCl pH 8.
10. Preservation buffer: PBS 1× with 0.02% NaN_3.

2.2 Antibody-Cross-Linking to Beads

1. 1% SDS.
2. Ultrapure water.
3. Beads: Protein A-Sepharose® 4B Conjugate.
4. 100 mM Tris–HCl pH 8.
5. 0.2 M Sodium Borate Buffer pH 9: Prepare solution A: dissolve 12.4 g of Boric acid in 1 L water. Prepare solution A: dissolve 12.4 g of Boric acid in 1 L water. In a new bottle mix 50 mL of solution A, 59 mL of solution B and 91 mL water to obtain 200 mL of 0.2 M Sodium Borate Buffer pH 9.
6. Purified W6-32 anti-pan HLA-I antibodies.
7. Purified IVA12 anti pan-HLA-II antibodies.
8. Dimethyl pimelimidate.
9. Ethanolamine solution: add 600 μL of ethanolamine to 50 mL of water, and adjust to pH 8 with HCl. Keep in the dark at room temperature (RT).
10. Preservation buffer: PBS 1× with 0.02% NaN_3.
11. Bio-Spin® disposable chromatography columns (Bio-Rad) with a stand.
12. NanoDrop.
13. Gel electrophoresis system.

2.3 Purification of HLA Class I and HLA Class II Binding Peptides

1. Flash frozen tumor tissues stored at −80 °C.
2. Lysis buffer: 0.25% sodium deoxycholate, 0.2 mM iodoacetamide (IAA), 1 mM EDTA, 1:200 Protease Inhibitors Cocktail (Sigma-Aldrich), 1 mM Phenylmethylsulfonylfluoride, 1% Octyl-beta-D glucopyranoside in PBS 1×. Prepare fresh (10 mL per 1 g of tissue). Keep on ice.
3. 100 mM Tris–HCl pH 8.
4. 100% ACN.
5. Wash solution A: 150 mM NaCl and 20 mM Tris–HCl pH 8. Keep on ice.
6. Wash solution B: 400 mM NaCl and 20 mM Tris–HCl pH 8. Keep on ice.
7. Wash solution C: 20 mM Tris–HCl pH 8. Keep on ice.
8. 1% TFA.
9. 0.1% TFA.
10. 0.1% TFA with 28% acetonitrile.

11. 0.1% TFA with 32% acetonitrile.
12. 0.1% TFA with 80% acetonitrile.
13. 2% ACN in 0.1% FA.
14. Positive Pressure-96 Processor (Waters) with extended self-made metal rods to accommodate the stacking of five 96-well plates (*see* **Note 2**).
15. 96-Well filtration plate (3 μm glass fiber and 10 μm polypropylene membrane, Seahorse Bioscience or alternatively 3 μm glass fiber and 25 μm polypropylene membrane from Agilent).
16. Sep-Pak tC18 96-well plate, 100 mg Sorbent per Well (Waters).
17. 96-Well "Collection" plates (2 mL per well, Waters).
18. 24-Well "Waste" plate (8 mL per well, Whatman).
19. 50 mL centrifuge tubes for the centrifugation of tissue samples.
20. ULTRA-TURRAX homogenizer (IKA or comparable equipment). Keep blade at 4 °C for tissue homogenization.
21. Laminar flow.
22. High-speed centrifuge.
23. Vacuum centrifuge.

2.4 Mass Spectrometry

1. LC-MS/MS. We use a Q Exactive HF mass spectrometer on-line coupled to nano-Easy 1200 UHPLC system fitted with Nanospray Flex™ source (Thermo Fisher Scientific).
2. Analytical column oven.
3. Analytical column with 8 μm tip opening and a dimension of 50 cm × 75 μm (new objectives).
4. ReproSil-Pur C18 1.9 μm particles 120 Å pore size resin (Dr. Maisch GmbH).

3 Methods

3.1 Preparation of Anti-HLA Cross-Linked Beads for IP of HLA Complexes

The protocol below describes the procedures for purification and cross-linking of antibodies sufficient for the IP of HLA-I and HLA-II complexes from 25 tissue samples of about 1 g each. The procedure can be scaled up or down according to the amount of available tissues.

3.1.1 Purification of Anti-HLA Antibodies from Hybridoma Growth Medium

5 mL of the hybridoma growth medium gives a yield of about 10–15 mg of W6-32 antibodies and 1–5 mg of IVA12 antibodies, respectively (*see* **Note 1**). Purified antibodies can be stored at −20 °C for future use. This procedure is performed on Bio-Rad columns and is solely based on gravity flow. Place the columns on a stand that is compatible with 15 mL collection tubes.

1. Label two separate Bio-Rad columns as "W6-32" and "IVA12," and wash well with 1% SDS and ultrapure water (*see* **Note 3**).
2. Add a final volume of 1 mL of beads per column. Allow the bead preservation solution to drain, and wash the beads with 10 mL of 100 mM Tris–HCl pH 8. Close the tip of the columns with the caps.
3. Load 5 mL of each of the growth medium containing the monoclonal antibodies into their respective columns, and let the medium flow through.
4. Wash the beads with 10 mL 100 mM Tris–HCl pH 8 and then with 10 mL of 20 mM Tris–HCl pH 8.
5. Elute the antibodies with serial elutions each of 1 mL using acetic acid 0.1 N pH 3 into Eppendorf Tubes containing 350 μL of 1 M Tris–HCl pH 8. Check that the pH is around 8. If needed, adjust pH of the eluted antibodies to pH 8 with 1 M Tris–HCl pH 8. Collect 3–4 elutions in total per antibody. Briefly vortex the Eppendorf Tubes.
6. Quantify the amount of antibodies in each tube using a Nano-Drop (*see* **Note 4**).
7. Wash the beads with 10 mL of 100 mM Tris–HCl pH 8 and then with 2 mL preservation buffer. Cover the beads with 2 mL of preservation buffer, and close the columns with the caps. Keep the columns at 4 °C for future use.

3.1.2 Chemical Cross-Linking of Anti-HLA Antibodies to Sepharose Beads

Sufficient amount of antibody-cross-linked beads should be generated to enable the parallel IP of your tissue samples of interest. Antibody-cross-linked beads can be stored at 4 °C for several months.

1. Into two separate Bio-Rad columns labeled as "W6-32-ProteinA" and "IVA12-ProteinA," add a final volume of 2 mL of fresh beads per column. Allow the bead preservation solution to drain, and wash the beads with 10 mL of 100 mM Tris–HCl pH 8. Close the tip of the columns with the caps.
2. Load 10 mg of each of the antibodies onto their correspondingly labeled columns. Close the columns with the upper caps and slowly rotate the columns at room temperature for 1 h. Any remaining unused antibodies can be stored at −20 °C for future use.
3. Remove caps and allow the liquid to drain. Wash the columns with 10 mL of 0.2 M Sodium Borate Buffer pH 9. Close the tips of the columns. Resuspend the beads with 2 mL of 0.2 M Sodium Borate Buffer pH 9. Transfer into new Eppendorf Tubes 30 μL of the resuspended beads from each column for SDS-gel analysis to evaluate the efficiency of the cross-linking.

4. Add 20.8 mg dimethyl pimelimidate (final concentration of 20 mM) directly into the column. Close the column completely and let rotate at room temperature for 30 min (*see* **Note 5**).
5. Open the upper caps and from each column transfer 30 μL of the beads into a new Eppendorf Tube. This is used for SDS-PAGE analysis to evaluate the efficiency of the cross-linking (*see* **Note 6**).
6. Open the tip and let the liquid flow through. Wash the beads with 5 mL of 0.2 M ethanolamine pH 8.
7. Close the tip and add 5 mL of ethanolamine solution. Close the columns and let rotate at room temperature for 2 h.
8. Open the caps. Allow the liquid to flow through. Wash the beads with 10 mL of preservation buffer. Cover the beads with 2 mL of preservation buffer and close the columns tightly. These can be kept at 4 °C for future use.

3.2 Purification of HLA Class I and HLA Class II Binding Peptides

3.2.1 Preparation of 96-Well Plates for Immunopurification

The amount of wells to be prepared for the IP procedure depends on the number of samples to be processed (*see* **Note 7**). 96-Well filtration plates' wells cannot be reused for other experiments. The described procedure is applicable for tissues and cell lines. We describe the protocol for HLA purification from tissue samples, and the procedure for cell lines is described in **Note 8**. "Pre-clear" plate containing Sepharose beads is additionally required for the depletion of endogenous antibodies from the tissue lysate. The positive Pressure-96 Processor is used in each step of the procedure to generate homogenous flow of liquid through the plates, unless stated otherwise. The processor's customized design requires the stacking of five plates to achieve proper flow through the plates. Therefore, some plates are used as a stand and must be added or removed depending on how many plates are required at each step of the purification. Exemplary schemes of the stacking of plates are shown in Fig. 1 for each step of the procedure.

1. Label distinct 96-well filtration plates as "Filter," "Pre-clear," "HLA-Ip," and "HLA-IIp." Label an 8 mL plate as "Waste" and a 2 mL plate as "Collection" (*see* **Note 9**).
2. Wash your assigned empty wells of the four filter plates separately by adding consecutively (put the plates on top of a "Waste" plate for each wash, and discard the liquid collected): 1 mL 100% CAN then 1 mL 0.1% TFA and 2 mL 100 mM Tris–HCl pH 8.
3. Load "W6-32-ProteinA" and "IVA12-ProteinA" cross-linked beads onto the "HLA-Ip" and "HLA-IIp" plates at a final bead volume of 75 μL in 100 mM Tris–HCl pH 8 per well, respectively. Collect the liquid in the "Waste" plate and discard it.

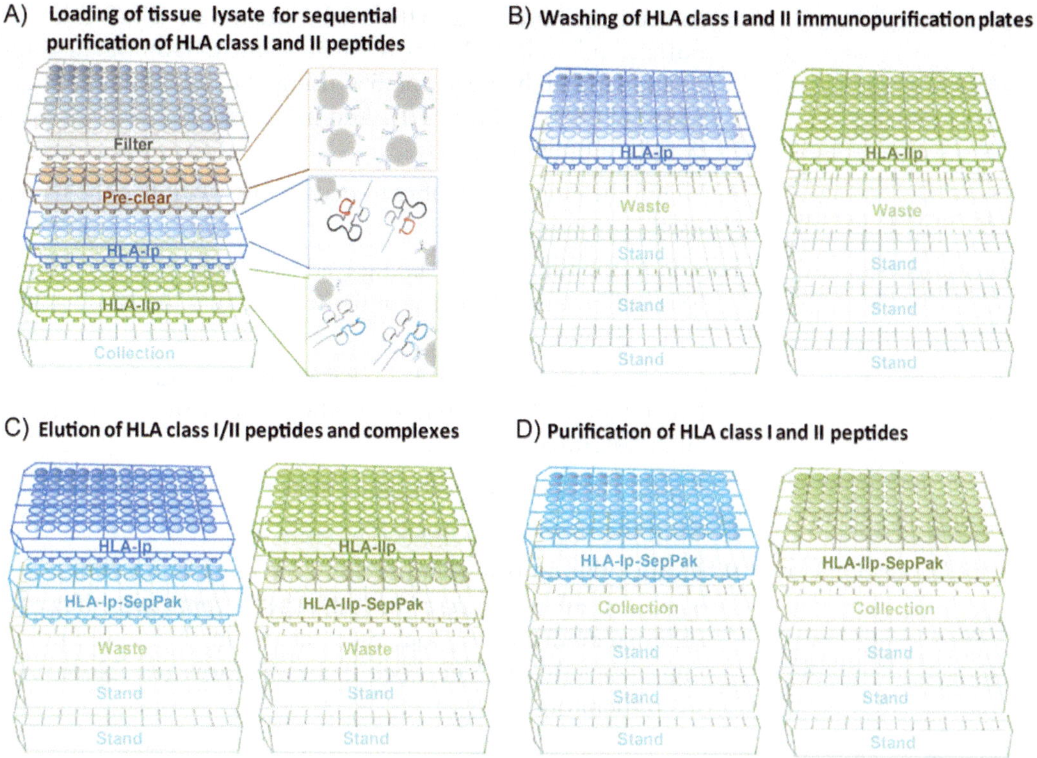

Fig. 1 (**a–d**) General overview of immuno-affinity based purification of HLA-I and HLA-II binding peptides from one tissue sample for mass spectrometry analysis. Tissue lysate is loaded on the "Filter" plate and will sequentially drop on the "Pre-clear," "HLA-Ip," and "HLA-IIp" for depleting autoantibodies and capturing HLA-I and HLA-IIp, respectively (**a**). "HLA-Ip" and "HLA-IIp" immunopurification plates containing the HLA-I and HLA-IIp are washed separately (**b**). HLA-I and HLA-IIp are acid eluted from "HLA-Ip" and "HLA-IIp" plates into "HLA-Ip- Sep-Pak" and "HLA-IIp-Sep-Pak" plates (**c**). HLA-I and HLA-IIp peptides are eluted separately from HLA class I and II complexes (**d**)

4. Add to each "Pre-clear" plate well 100 μL beads. Collect the liquid on the "Waste" plate and discard it.
5. Stack the plates from top to bottom as follows: (1) "Filter," (2) "Pre-clear," (3) "HLA-Ip," (4) "HLA-IIp," and (5) 2 mL "Collection" plate for collecting the lysate. (Fig. 1a, *see* **Note 9**).

3.2.2 Sample Preparation for Purification of HLA Class I and HLA Class II Peptides

Keep all tubes and solutions on ice during the sample preparation.

1. Place the ULTRA-TURRAX homogenizer inside a laminar flow in order to protect the user from aerosols that may be generated during the homogenization of the tissues.
2. Weigh the cryotubes containing the snap-frozen tissue and take note.
3. Process the tissues one at a time as follows: place the centrifuge tube in a cup filled with ice. With a pair of tweezers, transfer the

frozen tissue directly into the tube containing 1–2 mL cold lysis buffer, and wait 1–2 min to thaw slightly. Homogenize the tissue with high speed for 5 s using the ULTRA-TURRAX homogenizer (*see* **Note 10**). Add more lysis buffer if necessary to fully submerge the tissue.

4. Weigh the empty cryotubes to deduce the weight of the tissues itself.
5. Add to the tube the remaining cold lysis buffer (around 10 mL lysis buffer needed for 1 g of tissue), and mix the lysate gently every 10 min.
6. Disassemble the ULTRA-TURRAX blade, and wash it with first ethanol, then water. Wipe the blade with a paper towel and reassemble.
7. Repeat the above steps for your remaining tissue samples.
8. Keep the tubes on ice for 1 h.
9. Balance the centrifuge tubes and centrifuge at 51,200 × *g* at 4 °C for 50 min using the high-speed centrifuge. Transfer supernatant fractions from each sample in their correspondingly labeled new Safe-Lock Tubes/Falcons (*see* **Note 11**). Keep them on ice.

3.2.3 Sequential IP of HLA Class I and HLA Class II Peptides

For the steps that involve the use of the positive Pressure 96-well Processor, it is advisable not to exceed the pressure of 3 psi.

1. Load 2 mL of the cleared lysate from each of the samples onto the assigned wells of the “Filter” plate stacked on top of the “Pre-clear,” “HLA-Ip,” “HLA-IIp” and “Collection” plates (Fig. 1a, *see* **Note 8**).
2. Place the plates in the fridge at 4 °C, and let lysates flow by gravity through the “HLA-Ip” and “HLA-IIp” plates. Collect the depleted lysate and store at −20 °C for future use.
3. Once the passed lysate has been collected, add the rest of the lysate on top, 2 mL at a time. Repeat the procedure until all the lysate has passed through the plates.
4. Remove the plates from the fridge and place them on the bench. Discard the “Filter” and “Pre-clear” plates.
5. Place the “HLA-Ip” and “HLA-IIp” plates separately on top of a “Waste” plates in the positive pressure manifold as shown in Fig. 1b.
6. Wash the wells in each of the “HLA-Ip” and “HLA-IIp” plates with 4 times 2 mL of wash solution A, then with 4 times 2 mL of wash solution B, followed again by 4 times 2 mL of wash solution A, and lastly with 2 times 2 mL of wash solution C.

3.2.4 Purification of HLA-Bound Peptides

It is possible to use pressures slightly higher than 3 psi for the desalting steps as Sep-Pak tC18 96-well plates can be subjected to higher pressures.

1. Prepare two Sep-Pak tC18 96-well plates; one for HLA class I and one for HLA class II peptide samples. Label them accordingly as "HLA-Ip-Sep-Pak" and "HLA-IIp-Sep-Pak." Place "Waste" plates below the Sep-Pak plates to collect and discard the washes.
2. Wash the plates first once with 2 mL of 80% ACN in 0.1% TFA and thereafter twice with 2 mL of 0.1% TFA. Discard the solutions collected in the "Waste" plate.
3. Stack the "HLA-Ip" and "HLA-IIp" filtration plates on top of the "HLA-Ip-Sep-Pak" and "HLA-IIp-Sep-Pak" plates, respectively, as shown in Fig. 1c.
4. Elute the complexes by adding 200 μL 1% TFA to the assigned wells of the "HLA-Ip" and "HLA-IIp" plates.
5. Add another 300 μL 1% TFA to complete the elution.
6. Discard the "HLA-Ip" and "HLA-IIp" plates.
7. Wash each of the "HLA-Ip-Sep-Pak" and "HLA-IIp-Sep-Pak" plates twice with 2 mL of Sep-Pak C-18 wash solution.
8. Place the "HLA-Ip-Sep-Pak" plate on top of a new "Collection" plate, and elute the HLA-I binding peptides with 250 μL of 28% ACN in 0.1% TFA twice as shown in Fig. 1d.
9. Place the "HLA-IIp-Sep-Pak" plate on top of a new collection plate, and elute the HLA-II binding peptides with 250 μL of 32% ACN in 0.1% TFA twice as shown in Fig. 1d.
10. Transfer the elutions containing the peptides from each well of the "Collection" plate into correctly labeled Safe-Lock Tubes.
11. For further eluting the higher molecular weight proteins, *see* **Note 12**.
12. Completely dry down the Safe-Lock Tubes containing the peptides using vacuum centrifugation at 30 °C.
13. Resuspend the peptides in 10 μL 2% ACN in 0.1% FA and store at −20 °C until MS analysis.

3.3 Mass Spectrometry Analyses

This part of the protocol describes the analysis of HLA peptides using the Easy 1200 UHPLC system coupled online to a Q Exactive HF mass spectrometer, both from Thermo Fisher Scientific. Other comparable instruments can be used. Analytical column with 8 μm tip opening and a dimension of 50 cm × 75 μm may be self-packed with the ReproSil-Pur C18 1.9 μm particles having 120 Å pore size resin (Dr. Maisch GmbH, Ammerbuch-Entringen, Germany). The analytical column should be heated to 50 °C using a column oven due to its length. Make sure that the analytical column is clean, and measure a blank sample before the HLA peptide samples to exclude carry over from previously measured samples. We suggest the sequential injection of two technical replicates of 3 μL each. The remaining sample may be used in the future to validate targets of interest by spiking in isotopically heavy-labeled synthetic peptides. Alternatively, remaining samples may be used for further fractionation. Use the same MS settings for HLA class I and HLA II peptidomes, unless indicated otherwise.

1. Place 7 μL of each HLA peptide samples in the autosampler. Inject the first 3 μL of the first sample.
2. Apply a linear gradient of 2–30% of 80% ACN and 0.1% formic acid at a flow rate of 250 nL/min over 120 min for HLA class I and 90 min for HLA class II samples.
3. Suggested settings for the mass spectrometer are: MS scan range can be set to 300 to 1650 *m/z* with a resolution of 60,000 (200 *m/z*) and a target value of 3e6 ions. Data may be acquired with data-dependent "top10" method, which isolates the ten most intense ions and fragments them by higher-energy collisional dissociation (HCD) with an applied normalized collision energy of 27% and with an AGC target value of 1e5 with a maximum injection time of 120 ms and MS/MS resolution was 15,000 (200 *m/z*). For HLA class I peptides, in case of unassigned precursor ion charge states, or charge states of four and above, no fragmentation should be performed. For HLA class II peptides, in case of unassigned precursor ion charge states, or charge states of one or of five and above, no fragmentation should be performed. Dynamic exclusion of fragmented *m/z* values from further selection can be set for 20 s.
4. Inject again 3 μL of the first sample (technical duplicate).
5. Wash the system with two standard wash runs before loading the next biological sample.

4 Notes

1. Grow hybridoma cells in CELLine 350 or CELLine 1000 bioreactor flasks (Integra Biosciences), and collect the supernatant according to the manufacturer instructions. Spin the supernatant down at maximum speed using benchtop centrifuge to remove cell debris. Transfer supernatant containing the highly concentrated monoclonal antibodies into new tubes and store at −20 °C until use. After thawing the supernatant, centrifuge down again at maximum speed prior to use.
2. The two metal rods of the Positive Pressure-96 Processor should be extended by an additional extension of 11.5 cm

each (total length is 23 cm per rod) in order to accommodate the stacking of five 96-well plates. This should be done in advance at a local workshop.

3. Wash the Bio-Rad columns with 10 mL 1% SDS and 80 mL of water to remove possible contaminants.
4. Recovery and purity of antibodies may be estimated by loading 1% of each of the eluates on SDS-PAGE under denaturing conditions. The light and heavy chains of the antibodies should be visible.
5. Store dimethyl pimelimidate at −20 °C, and warm it to room temperature before use.
6. Add SDS sample loading buffer to the retained bead samples, heat at 95 °C for 5 min, and shortly spin down. Load 15 μL of the supernatant on an SDS-PAGE gel. Both the heavy and light chains of the antibodies should be visible in the samples before the cross-linking, while the heavy chains are not visible in the samples after cross-linking.
7. It is advisable to write down the corresponding well number for each sample.
8. For the immunoaffinity purification of HLA complexes from cell lines, typically 10^8 cells are used. Wash the cells with PBS, and after centrifugation, store the pellet of cells at −20 °C until use. Add lysis buffer at a concentration of 10^8 cells per mL. Add the cell lysates directly onto the "HLAI-p" plate stacked on the "HLAII-p" plate. As opposed to tissue samples, "Filter" and "Pre-clear" plates can be omitted for cell lines.
9. Tissues sometimes can contain a high quantity of fat, which cannot be removed even after extensive centrifugation. For this reason, it is advisable to add on top of the "Pre-clear" plate another empty 96-well filtration plate labeled as "Filter" plate as shown in Fig. 1a. This extra plate will help to remove the fat contained in the supernatant and will prevent clogging.
10. A longer homogenization might be needed depending on the tissue content. Generally, avoid prolonged homogenization as this leads to overheating of the tissues. Keep tubes sufficiently submerged on ice at all times.
11. The pellet formed during centrifugation can be kept at −20 °C or −80 °C for the extraction of DNA or RNA in the future, if required.
12. For further elution of the higher molecular weight proteins, place another collection plate, and elute the proteins with 500 μL of 80% ACN in 0.1% TFA. Pipette the protein solutions from each well of the collection plate into correctly labeled Safe-Lock Tubes. Completely dry down the Safe-Lock Tubes containing proteins using vacuum centrifugation at 30 °C.

Resuspend the proteins with PBS 1×. Analyze 10 μL of each elution by SDS-PAGE to evaluate the yield and the purity of the HLA complexes. Store remaining samples at −20 °C. The HLA-I heavy chain and the β2m should appear as 43 kDa and a 12 kDa bands, respectively. The two subunits of the HLA-II should appear as a broad band that is spread around the 28–30 kDa.

References

1. Neefjes J, Jongsma ML, Paul P, Bakke O (2011) Towards a systems understanding of MHC class I and MHC class II antigen presentation. Nat Rev Immunol 11(12):823–836. https://doi.org/10.1038/nri3084
2. Chong C, Marino F, Pak HS, Racle J, Daniel RT, Muller M, Gfeller D, Coukos G, Bassani-Sternberg M (2017) High-throughput and sensitive immunopeptidomics platform reveals profound IFNgamma-mediated remodeling of the HLA ligandome. Mol Cell Proteomics 17 (3):533–548. https://doi.org/10.1074/mcp.TIR117.000383
3. Pritchard AL, Hastie ML, Neller M, Gorman JJ, Schmidt CW, Hayward NK (2015) Exploration of peptides bound to MHC class I molecules in melanoma. Pigment Cell Melanoma Res 28(3):281–294. https://doi.org/10.1111/pcmr.12357
4. Jarmalavicius S, Welte Y, Walden P (2012) High immunogenicity of the human leukocyte antigen peptidomes of melanoma tumor cells. J Biol Chem 287(40):33401–33411. https://doi.org/10.1074/jbc.M112.358903
5. Bassani-Sternberg M, Pletscher-Frankild S, Jensen LJ, Mann M (2015) Mass spectrometry of human leukocyte antigen class I peptidomes reveals strong effects of protein abundance and turnover on antigen presentation. Mol Cell Proteomics 14(3):658–673. https://doi.org/10.1074/mcp.M114.042812
6. Dargel C, Bassani-Sternberg M, Hasreiter J, Zani F, Bockmann JH, Thiele F, Bohne F, Wisskirchen K, Wilde S, Sprinzl MF, Schendel DJ, Krackhardt AM, Uckert W, Wohlleber D, Schiemann M, Stemmer K, Heikenwalder M, Busch DH, Richter G, Mann M, Protzer U (2015) T cells engineered to express a T-cell receptor specific for glypican-3 to recognize and kill Hepatoma cells in vitro and in mice. Gastroenterology 149(4):1042–1052. https://doi.org/10.1053/j.gastro.2015.05.055
7. Weinschenk T, Gouttefangeas C, Schirle M, Obermayr F, Walter S, Schoor O, Kurek R, Loeser W, Bichler KH, Wernet D, Stevanovic S, Rammensee HG (2002) Integrated functional genomics approach for the design of patient-individual antitumor vaccines. Cancer Res 62(20):5818–5827
8. Singh-Jasuja H, Emmerich NP, Rammensee HG (2004) The Tubingen approach: identification, selection, and validation of tumor-associated HLA peptides for cancer therapy. Cancer Immunol Immunother 53 (3):187–195. https://doi.org/10.1007/s00262-003-0480-x
9. Bassani-Sternberg M, Barnea E, Beer I, Avivi I, Katz T, Admon A (2010) Soluble plasma HLA peptidome as a potential source for cancer biomarkers. Proc Natl Acad Sci U S A 107 (44):18769–18776. https://doi.org/10.1073/pnas.1008501107
10. Khodadoust MS, Olsson N, Wagar LE, Haabeth OA, Chen B, Swaminathan K, Rawson K, Liu CL, Steiner D, Lund P, Rao S, Zhang L, Marceau C, Stehr H, Newman AM, Czerwinski DK, Carlton VE, Moorhead M, Faham M, Kohrt HE, Carette J, Green MR, Davis MM, Levy R, Elias JE, Alizadeh AA (2017) Antigen presentation profiling reveals recognition of lymphoma immunoglobulin neoantigens. Nature 543(7647):723–727. https://doi.org/10.1038/nature21433
11. Kalaora S, Barnea E, Merhavi-Shoham E, Qutob N, Teer JK, Shimony N, Schachter J, Rosenberg SA, Besser MJ, Admon A, Samuels Y (2016) Use of HLA peptidomics and whole exome sequencing to identify human immunogenic neo-antigens. Oncotarget 7 (5):5110–5117. https://doi.org/10.18632/oncotarget.6960
12. Bassani-Sternberg M, Braunlein E, Klar R, Engleitner T, Sinitcyn P, Audehm S, Straub M, Weber J, Slotta-Huspenina J, Specht K, Martignoni ME, Werner A, Hein R, D HB, Peschel C, Rad R, Cox J, Mann M, Krackhardt AM (2016) Direct identification of clinically relevant neoepitopes presented on native human melanoma tissue by mass spectrometry. Nat Commun 7:13404. https://doi.org/10.1038/ncomms13404

13. Carreno BM, Magrini V, Becker-Hapak M, Kaabinejadian S, Hundal J, Petti AA, Ly A, Lie WR, Hildebrand WH, Mardis ER, Linette GP (2015) Cancer immunotherapy. A dendritic cell vaccine increases the breadth and diversity of melanoma neoantigen-specific T cells. Science 348(6236):803–808. https://doi.org/10.1126/science.aaa3828
14. Schumacher TN, Schreiber RD (2015) Neoantigens in cancer immunotherapy. Science 348 (6230):69–74. https://doi.org/10.1126/science.aaa4971
15. Mommen GP, Frese CK, Meiring HD, van Gaans-van den Brink J, de Jong AP, van Els CA, Heck AJ (2014) Expanding the detectable HLA peptide repertoire using electron-transfer/higher-energy collision dissociation (EThcD). Proc Natl Acad Sci U S A 111 (12):4507–4512. https://doi.org/10.1073/pnas.1321458111
16. Kowalewski DJ, Stevanovic S (2013) Biochemical large-scale identification of MHC class I ligands. Methods Mol Biol 960:145–157. https://doi.org/10.1007/978-1-62703-218-6_12
17. Loffler MW, Chandran PA, Laske K, Schroeder C, Bonzheim I, Walzer M, Hilke FJ, Trautwein N, Kowalewski DJ, Schuster H, Gunder M, Carcamo Yanez VA, Mohr C, Sturm M, Nguyen HP, Riess O, Bauer P, Nahnsen S, Nadalin S, Zieker D, Glatzle J, Thiel K, Schneiderhan-Marra N, Clasen S, Bosmuller H, Fend F, Kohlbacher O, Gouttefangeas C, Stevanovic S, Konigsrainer A, Rammensee HG (2016) Personalized peptide vaccine-induced immune response associated with long-term survival of a metastatic cholangiocarcinoma patient. J Hepatol 65(4):849–855. https://doi.org/10.1016/j.jhep.2016.06.027

Chapter 6

Identification of Immune Modulatory miRNAs by miRNA Enrichment via RNA Affinity Purification

Uta Sandy Tretbar, Michael Friedrich, Maria-Filothei Lazaridou, and Barbara Seliger

Abstract

Immune escape by cancer cells can be triggered by aberrant expression of immunological key players, which can be achieved by distinct molecular mechanisms including immune modulatory miRNAs. One suitable method to identify miRNAs that specifically target immune relevant molecules is the miRNA enrichment via RNA affinity purification method named miTRAP (miRNA trapping by RNA in vitro affinity purification). Here, we present a detailed protocol for construct preparation, RNA immobilization via MS2BP-MBP to beads, miRNA enrichment, and elution followed by analysis of the obtained miRNA candidates via qRT-PCR.

Key words miRNAs, RNA in vitro affinity purification, miTRAP, miRNA enrichment, Immune relevant

1 Introduction

One hallmark of cancer is the evasion of tumor cells from immune surveillance by various strategies [1]. Important mechanisms of immune evasion are, e.g., the aberrant expression of immune inhibitory molecules, such as the programmed death receptor 1 (PD-1) and its ligand PD-L1 and the nonclassical human leukocyte antigens (HLA)-G and (HLA)-E, and the impaired expression of the major histocompatibility complex (MHC) class I antigen processing and presenting machinery (APM) components, e.g., MHC class I heavy chain (HC), β_2-microglobulin (β_2-m), transporter associated with antigen processing (TAP) subunits, and the TAP-binding protein tapasin (tpn) (Fig. 1) [2].

The altered expression of these immune relevant genes could be due to posttranscriptional regulation mediated by microRNAs (miRNAs), which are termed immune modulatory miRNAs (im-miRNAs). While tumor suppressive miRNAs have been shown to induce the stimulation of the immune system, oncogenic

Yago Pico de Coaña (ed.), *Immune Checkpoint Blockade: Methods and Protocols*, Methods in Molecular Biology, vol. 1913,
https://doi.org/10.1007/978-1-4939-8979-9_6, © Springer Science+Business Media, LLC, part of Springer Nature 2019

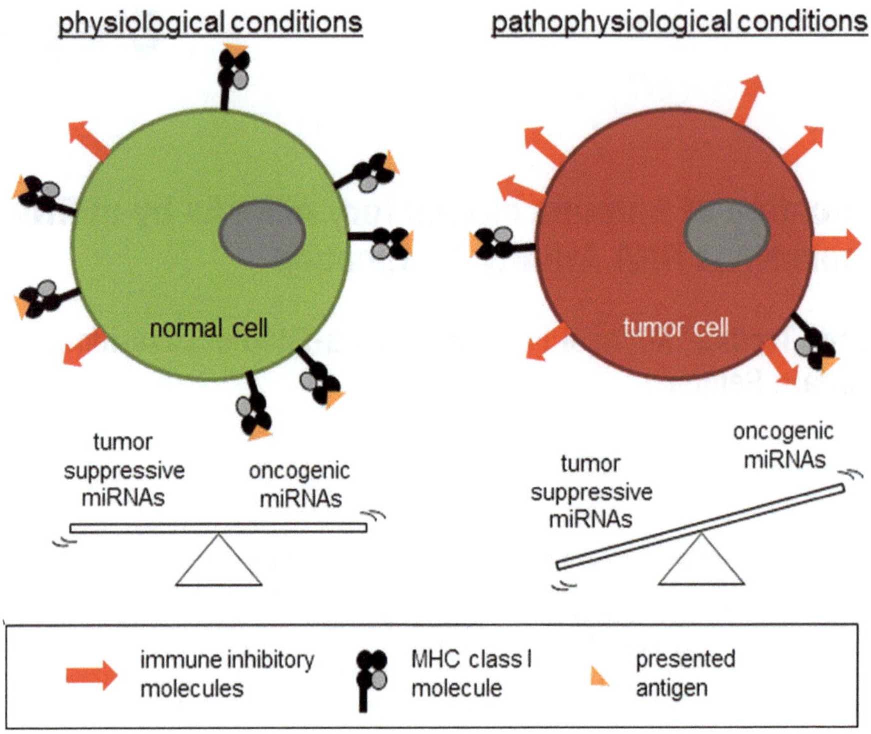

Fig. 1 The role of immune modulatory miRNAs under physiological and pathophysiological conditions

Table 1
Selection of immune escape relevant miRNAs and respective target genes

miRNA	Target mRNA	Reference
miR-9	β_2-m, TAP1, HLA-B, HLA-C	[5]
miR-20a	MICA/MICB	[6, 7]
miR-34a	PD-L1	[8]
miR-148a,b	HLA-C, HLA-G	[9, 10]
miR-152	HLA-G	[11]
miR-200	PD-L1	[12]

miRNAs determine immune suppression. In tumors, tumor suppressive miRNAs are often downregulated, and oncogenic miRNAs are upregulated leading to immune escape of the tumor cells (Fig. 1) [3]. A selection of already described im-miRNAs involved in immune evasion and their respective targets is shown in Table 1. One method used to identify such im-miRNAs is the miRNA trapping by RNA in vitro purification (miTRAP) method adapted from Braun and co-workers [4], which is refined for routinely use in our laboratory and presented here in detail.

2 Materials

All solutions are prepared with Millipore water (Merck Millipore, Burlington, MA, USA) and analytical grade reagents. Sterile plastic ware is used for all the procedures. Primers are purchased from Invitrogen (Carlsbad, CA, USA) and restriction enzymes from NEB (New England Biolabs, Ipswich, MA, USA).

2.1 Cloning Procedure

1. PCR components: Q5 DNA polymerase with corresponding 1x reaction buffer, dNTPs, oligonucleotides p01 and p02 (*see* Table 2).
2. Plasmid DNA pcDNA™ 3.1(+) (Invitrogen).
3. Restriction enzymes XhoI, ApaI, AflII.
4. Quick Ligation Kit (NEB).
5. Ultracompetent *E. coli* XL2 blue cells (Stratagene, La Jolla, CA, USA), genotype: *endA1 supE44 thi-1 hsdR17 recA1 gyrA96 relA1 lac* [F′ *proAB lacI*^{q}*ZΔM15* Tn*10* (Tet^r) Amy Cam^r].

2.2 RNA Preparation

1. *E. coli* dam$^-$/dcm$^-$ cells from NEB, genotype: *ara-14 leuB6 fhuA31 lacY1 tsx78 glnV44 galK2 galT22 mcrA dcm-6 hisG4 rfbD1 R(zgb210::Tn10)* Tet^S *endA1 rspL136* (Str^R) *dam13::Tn9* (Cam^R) *xylA-5 mtl-1 thi-1 mcrB1 hsdR2* (*see* **Note 1**).
2. NucleoBond Xtra Midi Kit for medium scale plasmid preparation (Macherey-Nagel).
3. Restriction enzymes PspOMI, ApaI, BclI.
4. PCR components: Taq polymerase with corresponding 1× reaction buffer, dNTPs, oligonucleotides p03 and p04 (Table 2).
5. QIAquick Gel Extraction Kit for purification of purification of digested plasmids (Qiagen).
6. In vitro transcription components: T7 RiboMAX™ Express Large Scale RNA Production System (Promega), reaction is supplemented with RNasin.
7. MEGAclear™ Kit for transcription reaction purification (Thermo Fisher).
8. Agarose gels.

2.3 Extract Preparation

1. 1× PBS, pH 7.4: 137 mM NaCl, 2.7 mM KCl, 10 mM Na_2HPO_4, 1.8 mM KH_2PO_4.
2. Cell lysis buffer: 20 mM Tris–HCl pH 7.5, 150 mM NaCl, 1.5 mM $MgCl_2$, 8.7% glycerol, 0.05% NP-40, protease inhibitor mix (1:200).

Table 2
List of oligonucleotides used in the procedure

RT = reverse transcription, SLP = stem-loop primer.

no.	name	sequence in 5′-3′ direction
p01	target-AflII fw	AAACTTAAG-target specific sequence
p02	target-XhoI rv	AAACTCGAG-target specific sequence
p03	T7 prom fw	TAATACGACTCACTATAGGGAG
p04	MS2 rv	GGTTTAAACGGGCCCAAAGACATG
p05	miR-222 RT SLP	GTCGTATCCAGTGCAGGGTCCGAGGTATTCGCACTGGATACGAC ACCCAG
p06	miR-222 qPCR fw	GCCCAGCTACATCTGGCTA
p07	miR-181b RT SLP	GTCGTATCCAGTGCAGGGTCCGAGGTATTCGCACTGGATACGAC ACCCAC
p08	miR-181b qPCR fw	GCCCAACATTCATTGCTGTCG
p09	miR-27a RT SLP	GTCGTATCCAGTGCAGGGTCCGAGGTATTCGCACTGGATACGAC GCGGAA
p10	miR-27a qPCR fw	CACGCATTCACAGTGGCTAAG
p11	SLP qPCR rv	CCAGTGCAGGGTCCGAGGTA

Fw Forward, *rv* Reverse, *RT* Reverse transcription, *SLP* Stem-loop primer

3. Cell storage buffer: Cell lysis buffer supplemented with 22 μg/mL heparin, 2 mM DTT, and 80 U RNasin.

2.4 Preparation of MS2BP-MBP Fusion Protein

1. LB medium.
2. IPTG (Isopropyl-β-D-thiogalactopyranosid).
3. *E. coli* BL21(DE3)pLysS cells (Thermo Fisher), genotype: F- *ompT hsdS*B (rBmB-) *gal dcm* (DE3)pLysS (Cam^R).
4. Amylose resin.
5. Binding buffer: 20 mM HEPES/KOH pH 7.9, 200 mM KCl, 1 mM EDTA, supplemented with one tablet Pierce Protease Inhibitor Mini Tablets, EDTA-free per 10 mL buffer.
6. Turbo DNase.
7. Elution buffer: binding buffer + 10 mM maltose.
8. Dialysis and storage buffer: cell lysis buffer (*see* Subheading 2.3).
9. Slide-A-Lyzer dialysis cassette (MWCO 3.500, Thermo Fisher).
10. Pierce BCA Protein Assay Kit (Thermo Fisher).

2.5 Protein and RNA-Binding Efficiency

1. Beads blocking buffer: cell lysis buffer, 250 μg/mL BSA, 20 μg/mL yeast tRNA.
2. Beads binding and wash buffer: cell lysis buffer, 11 μg/mL heparin.
3. RNA elution buffer: 15 mM maltose solution.
4. Protein sample buffer (4×): 187.7 mM Tris–HCl pH 6.8, 1.9 mM β-mercaptoethanol, 0.2 mM bromophenol blue.
5. RNA sample buffer, denaturing (3×): 10 mM Tris–HCl pH 7.6, 80% (v/v) formamide, 0.025% (w/v) xylene cyanole FF, 0.025% bromophenol blue.
6. SDS and denaturing PAA gels.
7. Rotation tube incubator.

2.6 MiRNA Enrichment Procedure

Additionally to components from Subheading 2.5:

1. Extract binding buffer: cell lysis buffer, 22 μg/mL heparin.
2. Proteinase K.
3. 7.5 M NH_4 acetate.
4. Phenol, chloroform, and isoamyl alcohol for RNA extraction.
5. Glycogen for RNA precipitation.

2.7 Western Blot

1. SDS gels.
2. 1× SDS running buffer: 25 mM Tris, 200 mM glycine, 0.1% SDS.
3. 1× transfer buffer: SDS running buffer, 10% methanol.
4. Nitrocellulose blotting membrane (GE Healthcare, Chalfont St Giles, GB).

5. Antibodies: anti-argonaute 2 (Abcam, Cambridge, GB), anti-maltose-binding protein (Abcam), anti-beta actin (Sigma, St. Louis, MO, USA), anti-mouse IgG HRP-linked (Cell Signaling, Cambridge, GB), anti-rabbit HRP-linked IgG (Cell Signaling).

2.8 MiRNA Analysis

1. First-strand cDNA synthesis kit.
2. miRNA-specific stem-loop and forward primers p05-10 (Table 2).
3. Sensoquest Thermocycler.
4. 2× SYBR green qPCR master mix.
5. Biorad CFX Connect Real-Time Cycler.

3 Methods

All steps are carried out at room temperature unless indicated otherwise. Use sterile, free of DNA, DNase/RNase, PCR inhibitors, ATP, and pyrogens/endotoxin tips and 1.5 mL tubes.

3.1 Construct Preparation

For efficient immobilization of bait RNA on beads, the MS2 tagging technique based on the interaction of the MS2 bacteriophage coat protein and specific RNA stem-loop structures from the phage genome is used [13]. Therefore, the DNA sequence of the target RNA of interest is cloned upstream of the coding sequence for two MS2 stem-loop structures (Fig. 2). Target sequences can be the 3′ untranslated region (UTR) of a gene, the coding region (CDS), the 5′ UTR as well as long noncoding RNAs (*see* **Note 2**).

1. The target sequence of interest is amplified in a standard PCR reaction with target-specific primers carrying overhangs with restriction recognition sites (p01, p02).
2. The pcDNA3.1(+) vector carrying a tandem repeat of the MS2 stem-loop motif downstream of a T7 promoter sequence and the target PCR product are digested with restriction enzymes such as AflII and XhoI according to the manufacturer's recommendation (*see* **Note 3**).
3. After cleanup of the digestion reaction, insert and vector are ligated using the Quick Ligation Kit.
4. *E. coli* XL2 blue cells are transformed with the ligation reactions.
5. Cloning success is tested using colony PCR.
6. Correct insertion of the target sequence of interest between T7 promoter and the two MS2 stem-loop motifs is verified by DNA sequencing.

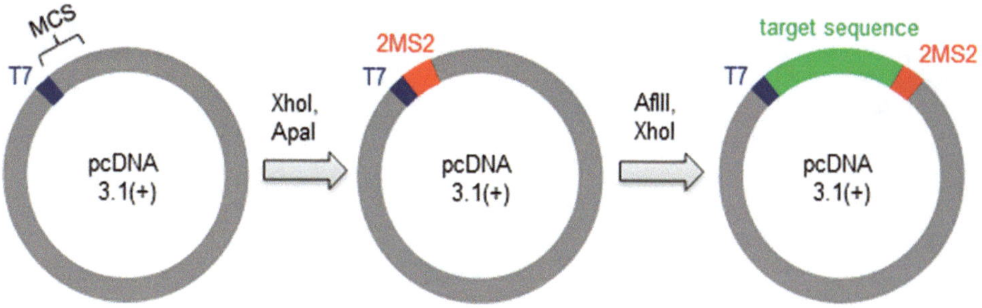

Fig. 2 Cloning strategy. The vector backbone is the pcDNA3.1(+) plasmid (gray) carrying a T7 promoter sequence (dark blue) upstream of the multiple cloning site (MCS). Using the restriction enzymes XhoI and ApaI, a tandem repeat of the MS2 stem-loop motif was inserted into the MCS (two MS2, red). The constructs are generated by insertion of a sequence of interest (green) upstream of the two MS2 loops using restriction enzymes that do not cut in the desired sequence, such as AflII and XhoI

3.2 RNA Preparation

For RNA preparation, the bacteriophage T7 RNA polymerase system is used. The polymerase recognizes its cognate promoter region in the DNA template and catalyzes RNA synthesis in 5′–3′ direction [14].

There are two ways to prepare the DNA template for in vitro transcription: linearization of the plasmid DNA (pDNA) or generation of a PCR product.

3.2.1 Linearization of the pDNA

1. *E. coli* dam^-/dcm^- cells are transformed with the pDNA carrying either the sequence of interest or only the two MS2 loops (*see* **Note 4**), and plasmid DNA is prepared using the NucleoBond Xtra kit (Macherey-Nagel).
2. 30 μg of purified pDNA are digested with PspOMI (or ApaI or BclI) in 1× cut smart buffer overnight at 37 °C (BclI requires Buffer 3.1 and 50 °C) (Fig. 3a).
3. Digested pDNA is purified using gel extraction with the QIAquick kit.
4. 10 μg of purified pDNA serve as template for the in vitro transcription reaction.

3.2.2 PCR Product Generation

1. Using the pDNA prepared in Subheading 3.1 as a template, a standard PCR with the forward primer p03 annealing to the T7 promoter and the reverse primer p04 partially annealing to the MS2 loops and partially to the vector backbone is performed (Fig. 3b).
2. PCR products are purified using the QIAquick kit.
3. 1 μg of purified PCR product serves as template for the in vitro transcription reaction.

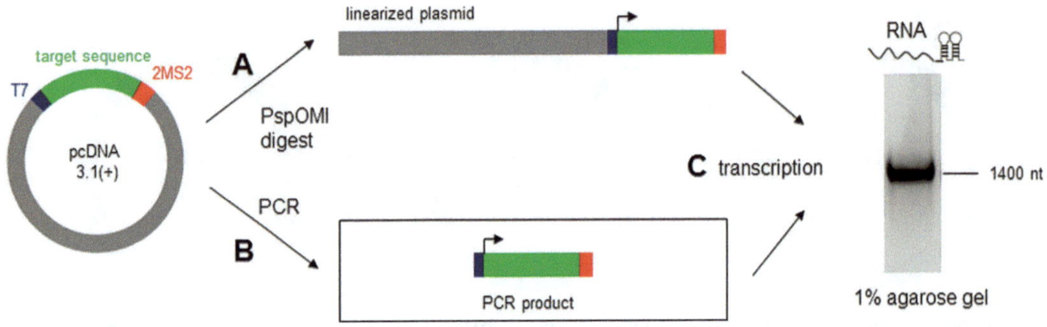

Fig. 3 Transcription procedure. The DNA template for the in vitro transcription reaction (C) can be generated either by (A) digestion of the plasmid DNA or (B) performing a PCR reaction. To linearize the pDNA, a restriction enzyme directly cutting downstream of the MS2 loops such as PspOMI or ApaI can be used

3.2.3 Transcription Reaction

1. Transcription of the target sequence of interest coupled to two MS2 loops or the two MS2 loops alone is performed using the RiboMax T7 Large Scale transcription kit according to the manufacturer's recommendations overnight at 37 °C.
2. The next day, the template DNA is removed by addition of 1 U RQ DNase I (provided with the transcription kit) per 1 μg DNA for 10 min at 37 °C.
3. Transcription reaction is analyzed by agarose gel electrophoresis (Fig. 3c, *see* **Note 5**) and purified using the MEGAclear kit according to the manufacturer's protocol.
4. The concentration of the RNA is determined using a TECAN Infinite 200 Pro microplate reader detecting the absorption at 260 nm. The molarity of the RNA is calculated using the following equation:

$$\text{RNA } [\text{pmol}/\mu L] = \frac{\text{RNA } [\text{ng}/\mu L] \times 1000}{\text{MW(RNA)}}$$

MW (RNA) = number of nucleotides × 325 g/mol (=average MW of nucleotides).

3.3 Extract Preparation

1. Harvest 1 × 10^7 cells of your desired cell line and wash pellet 3× with 1× PBS (*see* **Note 6**). The amount of cells is sufficient for one target RNA + one MS2 control + one beads control + one RNA input preparation.
2. Resuspend the cells in 2 mL cell lysis buffer and incubate 15 min on ice.
3. Spin the lysate for 10 min at 11,000 × *g* and 4 °C, and transfer the supernatant into a new tube, keep on ice!
4. Keep 500 μL of the supernatant for RNA input preparation (*see* Subheading 3.6) on ice.

5. To the remaining 1.5 mL lysate, add an equal amount of cell storage buffer.
6. 1 mL supplemented cell lysate is required per reaction and kept on ice until use in the miRNA enrichment step (*see* **Note 7**).

3.4 Preparation of MS2BP-MBP Fusion Protein

Expression and affinity purification via amylose resin and gravity flow are adopted from and optimized according to Jurica and co-workers [15] as well as the pMal fusion and purification system from NEB (#E8200S, manualE8200).

3.4.1 Expression of MS2BP-MBP Fusion Protein

1. *E. coli* BL21(DE3)pLysS cells are transformed with the pMalC vector carrying the MS2BP-MBP fusion gene.
2. A 5 mL pre-culture LB medium + ampicillin (100 μg/mL) + chloramphenicol (25 μg/mL) is inoculated with one colony from the retransformation (*see* **Note 8**) and incubated in a shaker overnight at 37 °C and 230 rpm.
3. The next day, 500 mL LB medium + ampicillin (100 μg/mL) + chloramphenicol (25 μg/mL) are inoculated with the 5 mL pre-culture (1 mL pre-culture per 100 mL medium).
4. The cells are incubated in the shaker 37 °C and 230 rpm until they reach an optical density OD_{600} of 0.6–0.8 (bacteria are in exponential phase then).
5. Take a sample prior to induction, and keep it in freezer until the gel run.
6. Add 1 mM IPTG to induce MS2BP-MBP protein expression from the plasmid (*see* **Note 9**).
7. Induce expression for 3 h with IPTG at 37 °C.
8. Take a sample after the induction, and analyze it on a 12% SDS gel for overexpression. A prominent band at 54 kDa should appear after induction with IPTG (Fig. 4a).
9. Collect the cells by centrifugation and either directly proceed with cell lysis or keep cell pellet at −80 °C until further use.

3.4.2 Affinity Purification of MS2BP-MBP Fusion Protein

1. If necessary, thaw cell pellet on ice.
2. Resuspend the pellet in 5 mL resuspension buffer and directly proceed with sonication.
3. Use microtip for solutions up to 15 mL; larger volumes require bigger tip.
4. Sonicate cells with a power level of 70% with a 15 s pulse, pause 30 s, and repeat this cycle 5 times.
5. Add 10 U Turbo DNase, and let sit for 30 min on ice.
6. Separate cell debris from the soluble fraction that contains MS2BP-MBP with a centrifugation step for 30 min at 4 °C and 21,000 × *g*.

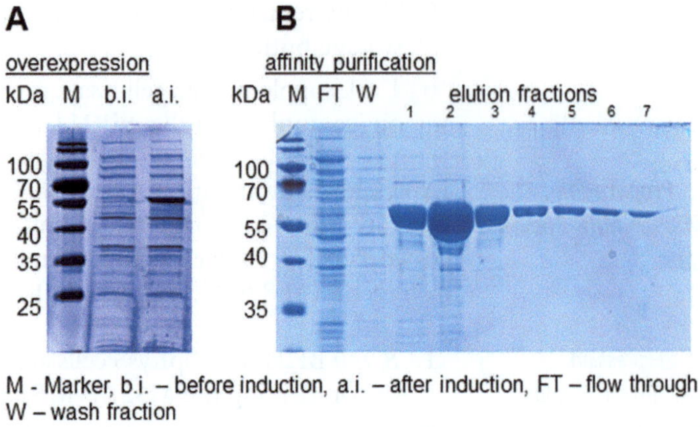

Fig. 4 MS2BP-MBP fusion protein preparation. SDS-PAGE analysis showing the overexpression and RNA affinity purification of MS2BP-MBP fusion protein. The expected size of the fusion protein is 54 kDa. (**a**) After induction with IPTG (a.i.), an additional prominent band appeared in comparison to the lysate before IPTG induction (b.i.) at around 55 kDa indicating solid expression of the MS2BP-MBP fusion protein. (**b**) Column flow through (FT) and wash fraction (W) do not contain considerable amounts of MS2BP-MBP indicating stable binding to the amylose resin. MS2BP-MBP was successfully eluted from the column in seven 1 mL fractions. Elution fractions 3–7 were specified as pure enough for subsequent dialysis

7. Transfer the supernatant to a novel tube and keep chilled on ice, and take pellet and supernatant sample for gel run (*see* **Note 10**).
8. Prepare column with amylose resin (*see* **Note 11**). From now on work on ice or in the cold room.
9. Fill the empty column with 2 mL of amylose resin slurry.
10. Remove the storage buffer via gravity flow.
11. Wash the column with 5 volumes of binding buffer (10 mL) (*see* **Note 12**).
12. Load the soluble fraction containing the MS2BP-MBP onto the column.
13. Collect and keep the flow through in case the protein does not bind and for SDS-PAGE analysis.
14. Wash the column with 6 volumes of binding buffer (12 mL), keep wash fraction for SDS-PAGE analysis.
15. Elute the MS2BP-MBP with a total volume of 7 mL of elution buffer → collect 1 mL elution fractions, and keep fractions for SDS-PAGE analysis and dialysis.
16. Prepare flow through, and wash and elute step samples for gel run (*see* **Note 13**):

(a) 3 μL flow through + 17 μL water + 5 μL SDS load → load 25 μL.

(b) 3 μL wash + 17 μL water + 5 μL SDS load → load 25 μL.

(c) 3 μL elution + 17 μL water + 5 μL SDS load → load 25 μL.

17. Combine elution fractions containing pure MS2BP-MBP fusion protein (Fig. 4b) for dialysis against cell lysis buffer.
18. Dialyze overnight at 4 °C with 600 mL of cell lysis buffer using a Slide-A-Lyzer cassette. The next day change the buffer and dialyze again for 4 h.
19. Determine the concentration of the protein using a BCA assay kit.
20. Prepare aliquots, flash freeze with liquid nitrogen, and store protein at −20 °C.

3.5 Protein and RNA-Binding Efficiency

To check the functionality of the MS2BP-MBP fusion protein for amylose beads and RNA binding, immobilization of MS2BP-MBP on the beads is analyzed. Subsequently, the efficiency of RNA binding to the fusion protein is determined for each construct.

Unless indicated otherwise, amylose beads are always separated from solutions by centrifugation in a bench top centrifuge for 15 s at full speed and room temperature. The supernatant is removed by pipetting. Incubation of beads and solutions is carried out in a rotation tube incubator at 30 rpm.

3.5.1 Protein Immobilization on Amylose Resin

1. Use 25 μL of the amylose resin per reaction, which corresponds to 55 μL slurry (55 μL slurry for 1 reaction, 110 μL for two reactions, etc.).
2. Completely remove the storage ethanol.
3. Wash the beads 1× with 0.5 mL of cell lysis buffer.
4. Add again 0.5 mL of cell lysis buffer, and if applicable distribute the combined reactions into separate tubes, spin samples, and remove the wash buffer completely.
5. Incubate the beads with 0.5 mL cell lysis buffer + 0, 10, 50, 100, or 200 pmol of MS2BP-MBP for 30 min.
6. After MS2BP-MBP immobilization, wash the beads 1× with cell lysis buffer.
7. Elute the protein from the beads by adding 25 μL of protein sample buffer.
8. Incubate for 5 min at 95 °C, spin down the beads, and analyze 20 μL of the supernatant in a 12% SDS gel (Fig. 5a).

3.5.2 RNA Immobilization on MS2BP-MBP Loaded Amylose Beads

1. Immobilize 200 pmol MS2BP-MBP per reaction on the amylose beads according to **steps 1–5** in Subheading 3.5.1. Reactions are still combined in that step.

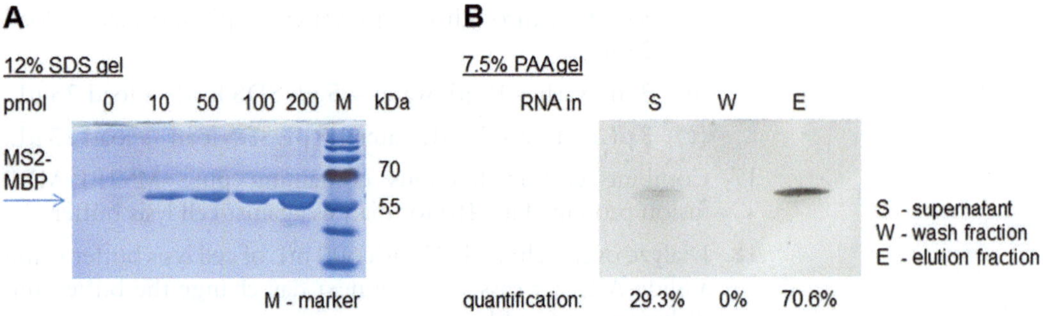

Fig. 5 Binding test for MS2BP-MBP and RNA. (**a**) The more protein was added for immobilization, the more was eluted from the beads. 200 pmol of the fusion protein was chosen to be the optimum amount for coupling RNA to the beads. (**b**) Analysis of the individual fractions of the RNA immobilization shows the most prominent band in the elution fraction. Quantification of the bands demonstrates a ca. 70% binding efficiency for the example target RNA of interest

2. After MS2BP-MBP immobilization, remove unbound protein and buffer completely.
3. Add 0.5 mL of beads blocking buffer, and incubate for 30 min.
4. In the meantime, heat the target RNA for 5 min at 65 °C and cool down at room temperature.
5. After the blocking step, wash beads 3× with beads wash buffer and distribute the beads equally into separate tubes according to the required number of reactions.
6. Immobilize 10 pmol of the target RNA in beads binding buffer + 1 μL RNasin for 1 h.
7. After RNA immobilization, keep the supernatant to check for unbound RNA.
8. Wash beads 1× with beads wash buffer, and keep the wash fraction.
9. Elute the RNA using 150 μL of RNA elution buffer by rotating the samples for 10 min.
10. Repeat the elution step and combine the elution fractions.
11. Perform NH_4-acetate precipitation and phenol/chloroform extraction of the eluted RNA (described more detailed in Subheading 3.6.3).
12. Perform ethanol precipitation of the supernatant (S) and wash (W) fraction as well as the eluted RNA (E). Take up the pellets in 10 μL RNase-free water.
13. Analyze 5 μL of each fraction (S, W and E) in a 7.5% denaturing polyacrylamide (PAA) gel containing 8 M urea.
14. Quantify the bands for binding efficiencies using ImageJ software [16] (Fig. 5b).

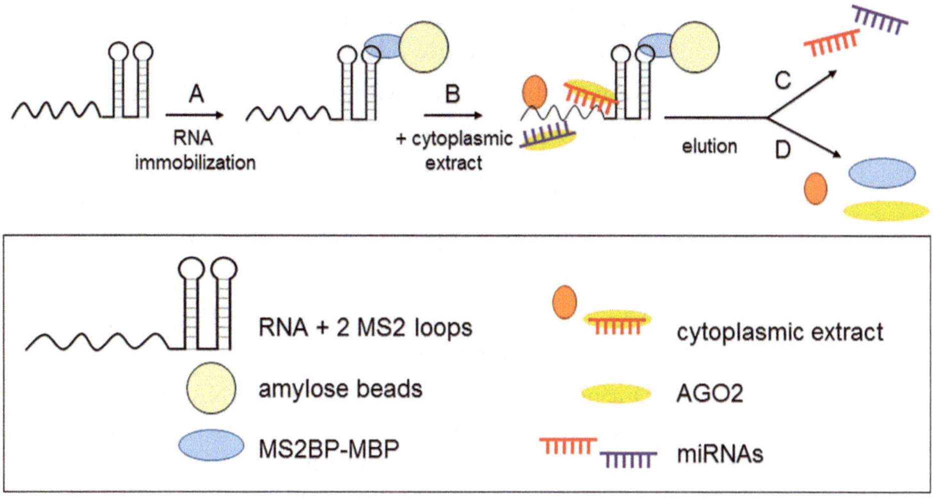

Fig. 6 Schematic of the miRNA enrichment procedure. After immobilization of the target RNA + two n MS2 stem-loops via MS2BP-MBP on amylose beads, cytoplasmic extract is incubated with the target RNA of interest. RNAs and proteins are separately eluted from the beads for downstream analyses, such as small RNA sequencing, qPCR, and Western blot

3.6 miRNA Enrichment Procedure

According to Subheading 3.5, amylose beads are always separated from solutions by centrifugation in a bench top centrifuge. Spinning steps occur for 15 s at 11,000 × *g* and room temperature. The supernatant is removed by pipetting. Incubation of beads and solutions is carried out in a rotation tube incubator at approximately 30 rpm.

After coupling of the MS2BP-MBP anchor for target RNA immobilization on the amylose beads, miRNAs are enriched on the target RNAs by incubating with cell extract from cells of interest. One set of miTRAP reactions consists of x target RNAs of interest, one MS2 only control (in vitro transcript of two MS2 stem-loops is immobilized as background control), and one bead control (no RNA was immobilized as background control) for one type of cell extract. If you use different cell extracts, MS2 only and beads control are needed for each type of extract! An overview of the entire procedure is shown in Fig. 6. Work at room temperature. Keep all the reagents on ice, except for the proteinase K at room temperature. If it is not required to check for Argonaute 2 (AGO2) via protein elution and you only want to elute RNA from your target RNA, use half the volume of all the reagents (e.g., amylose beads, cell lysis buffer, BSA, tRNA, RNA, cell lysate). All the following steps are performed on ice.

3.6.1 RNA Immobilization

1. Mix gently the amylose resin in order to resuspend them in the storage ethanol. Use 50 μL of the amylose beads per reaction, which is equivalent to 110 μL slurry. Combine the beads for one set of miTRAP reactions into one 1.5 mL tube. Separate

beads from storage solution, and remove the supernatant completely (*see* **Note 14**).

2. Wash the beads twice with 0.5 mL cell lysis buffer.
3. Add 0.5 mL cell lysis buffer and 400 pmol of MS2BP-MBP fusion protein per miTRAP reaction and immobilize the protein for 30 min on the turning wheel (*see* **Note 15**).
4. After MS2BP-MPB immobilization, remove the supernatant completely.
5. Add 1 mL beads blocking buffer, and rotate the samples for 30 min (*see* **Note 16**).
6. During sample rotation, heat the RNA (50 pmol RNA per miTRAP reaction) for 5 min at 65 °C (*see* **Note 17**), and let it cool down at room temperature.
7. After the beads blocking step, remove the supernatant completely.
8. Wash the beads three times with 0.5 mL cell lysis buffer. With the last wash step, equally distribute the samples into respective tubes for each miTRAP reaction.
9. Add 50 pmol target RNA and 10–50 pmol two MS2 loop RNA only as control reaction in 0.5 mL beads binding buffer and 40 U RNasin (*see* **Note 18**). One tube without RNA serves as background control. Immobilize the RNA on the beads for 1 h on the turning wheel.

3.6.2 miRNA Enrichment Procedure

1. During the RNA immobilization on the amylose beads, prepare the extract as described in Subheading 3.3.
2. After the 1 h rotation, remove the supernatant completely.
3. Wash the beads twice with 0.5 mL beads wash buffer, and remove the buffer completely.
4. Add 1 mL of the prepared extract to each tube and incubate for 30 min on the turning wheel.
5. During the 30 min rotation, digest 500 μL of the cell lysate with 100 μg/mL proteinase K at 50 °C for 15 min. Keep the digested extract as the input control on ice until phenol/chloroform RNA extraction.
6. After the 30 min rotation, remove the supernatant completely.
7. Wash the beads four times with 0.5 mL beads wash buffer, and remove the buffer completely. With the last wash step, distribute equally each miTRAP reaction tube into two tubes for RNA and protein elution, respectively.

3.6.3 RNA Elution

1. Add 150 μL RNA elution buffer, resuspend the beads, and rotate the samples for 10 min on the turning wheel at room temperature.

2. Centrifuge the samples at 11,000 × *g* for 15 s, and transfer the first elution fraction into new tubes. Keep the tubes on ice.
3. Repeat the elution step one more time, and combine the two elution fractions.
4. For the miTRAP elutions and the input control sample, perform NH_4 acetate precipitation by mixing gently 2 volumes of RNA solution with 1 volume of 7.5 M NH_4 acetate.
5. Perform phenol/chloroform RNA extraction by adding 300 μL phenol and 300 μL chloroform/isoamyl alcohol (in ratio 24:1, v/v) to the RNA solution (*see* **Note 19**). Vortex the tubes for 10 s, and centrifuge them at 2500 × *g* for 2 min at room temperature. Transfer the supernatant aqueous phase into a new tube.
6. Add 200 μL nuclease-free H_2O to the phenol/chloroform/isoamyl alcohol mixture in order to extract any remaining RNA. Vortex the tubes for 15 s, and centrifuge them at 2500 × *g* for 2 min at room temperature. Transfer the supernatant aqueous phase into the same tube.
7. Add 1 volume isopropanol and 10–20 μg RNase-free glycogen to precipitate the RNA (*see* **Note 20**).
8. Store the samples at least 20 min at −20 °C or, optionally, overnight.
9. Centrifuge the samples at 11,000 × *g* for 15 min at 4 °C, and remove the supernatant.
10. Wash the pellets once with 1 mL 70% ethanol. Centrifuge the samples at 11,000 × *g* for 15 min at 4 °C and remove the supernatant.
11. Resuspend gently the pellet of miTRAP eluate samples in 10 μL nuclease-free H_2O and the pellet of input control samples in 32 μL nuclease-free H_2O. Store the samples at −80 °C.

3.6.4 Protein Elution

1. For protein elution, add 25 μL protein sample buffer (incl. 10% beta-mercaptoethanol) to the miTRAP reactions.
2. Additionally, prepare 0.5%, 2%, and 5% dilution series of the cell lysate as input controls.
3. Heat the samples for 5 min at 95 °C for denaturation of the proteins.
4. Centrifuge the samples at 11,000 × *g* for 15 s and load 20 μL of the supernatant and all of the cell lysate dilution series on a 10% SDS-PAA gel.

3.7 Western Blotting

Functional miRNAs are necessarily associated with one of the four human Argonaute proteins (AGO1-4) to form the minimal RNA-induced silencing complex (RISC). Since the majority of

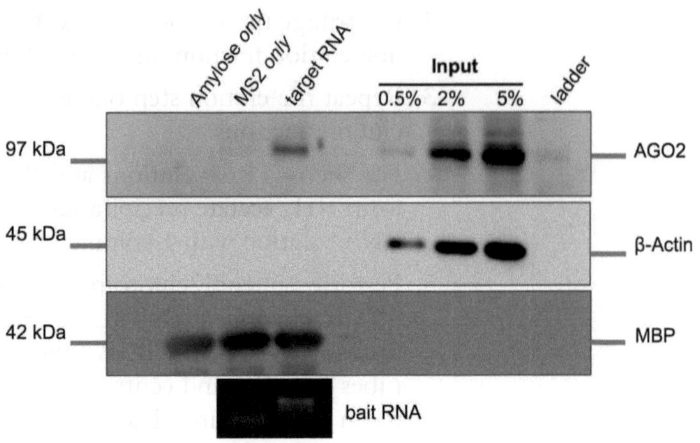

Fig. 7 Western blot analysis to check for AGO2 presence and PAA gel analysis to check for target RNA integrity after the miRNA enrichment procedure. An AGO2 (Argonaute 2) signal is detected for the cell lysate input control samples as well as on the target RNA indicating miRNA delivery and binding to the target RNA by AGO2. No AGO2 signal was detected in the amylose beads control. MiRNAs detected in the MS2 only eluate is regarded as background binding. Unspecific protein binding to the beads can be excluded by the lack of a β-Actin signal on the beads and target RNA. A signal for the maltose-binding protein (MBP) part of the MS2BP-MBP fusion protein is detected in the eluates but not in the cell extract. The lower panel represents a denaturing agarose gel showing the integrity of the target (bait) RNAs after miRNA enrichment procedure

miRNAs is incorporated into AGO2 [17], Western blot-based detection of co-purified AGO2 in miTRAP eluates indirectly indicates the presence of miRNAs. In addition, the specificity of the method can be monitored using a non-binding control such as β-actin (Fig. 7).

1. Separate co-purified proteins, and input samples according to their molecular weight by SDS gel electrophoresis.
2. Transfer proteins in a Trans-Blot cell (Bio-Rad, Hercules, CA, USA) for 16 h (10 V/100 mA) to a suitable membrane by wet electroblotting ("tank blot").
3. Block the membrane with 5% nonfat-dried milk diluted in TBS-T for 1 h at room temperature. Wash the membrane with TBS-T for 10 min.
4. Incubate the membrane with the primary antibody (e.g., anti-AGO2, 1:1000 in 5% BSA, TBS-T) overnight at 4 °C. Wash 3 times for 10 min with TBS-T.
5. Incubate membrane with HRP-coupled secondary antibody (e.g., anti-rabbit, 1:1000 in 5% nonfat-dried milk, TBS-T) for 2 h. Wash 3 times for 10 min with TBS-T.
6. Use a chemiluminescent substrate, and capture the signal with an X-ray film or a CCD camera imaging device.

3.8 miRNA Analysis

The eluates obtained from the miRNA enrichment procedure may be used to identify novel miRNAs targeting gene of interest. A "holistic" identification of co-purified miRNAs can either be achieved by high-throughput sequencing of short RNAs (miRNA-Seq) or using the microarray technology. In addition, several tools for in silico miRNA target prediction, like TargetScan [18], PITA [19], and miRanda [20], have been developed. In order to verify the resulting data in miTRAP eluates, specific miRNAs can be quantified by qRT-PCR.

1. Prepare first-strand cDNA reaction according to manufacturers' instructions (*see* **Note 21**). Use 1/5th of the miTRAP eluate or 1/50th of input RNA for reverse transcription. As reported by Kramer [21], a final concentration of 1 nm for miRNA-specific stem-loop primer can give specific results. The possibility of multiplexing stem-loop primers needs to be analyzed for individual assays.
2. Reactions are incubated for 30 min at 16 °C, 30 min at 42 °C, and 5 min at 85 °C and then held at 4 °C [22].
3. Prepare qRT-PCR reactions according to manufacturers' instructions (*see* **Note 22**). Use 1/10th of the first-strand cDNA reaction as input.
4. Run qRT-PCR at standard conditions:

1 cycle	10 min 95 °C
40 cycles	30 s 95 °C
	30 s 60 °C

5. Data analysis: co-purification of miRNAs can be specified as miTRAP ratio [4], indicating the ratio of miRNA abundance in the miTRAP eluate versus the input determined by the ΔC_t-method. Alternatively, enrichment of miRNAs can be assessed using the ratio of miRNA abundance in the miTRAP eluate from a target RNA versus MS2 only control (Fig. 8).

4 Notes

1. *E. coli* dam$^-$/dcm$^-$ cells are methylation-deficient bacteria. PspOMI is a methylation-sensitive restriction enzyme, and its activity may be blocked by CpG methylation.
2. It is recommended to use constructs of about 1500 bp maximum length to ensure efficient in vitro transcription. The longer the target sequences, the lower the amount of RNA after in vitro transcription. However, if you have longer constructs, you can test the transcription efficiency. If you receive

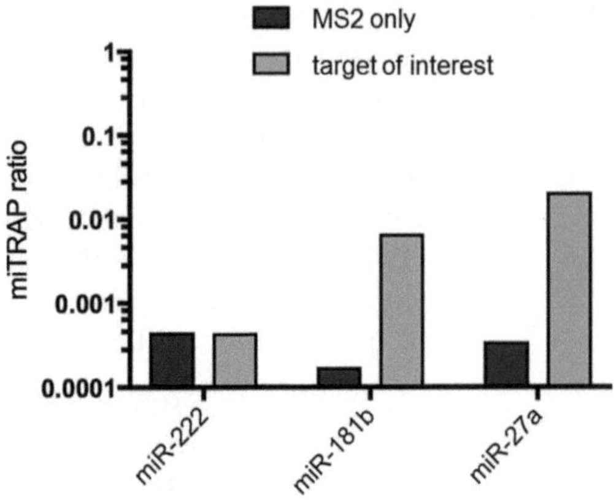

Fig. 8 Quantification of miRNAs in miTRAP eluates. Bar graph showing the miTRAP ratio of three different miRNAs. Given that the input value is 1, the bars show the enrichment of the respective miRNA on the MS2 only RNA (dark gray) in comparison to the used target RNA (light gray). For miR-222 no specific binding to the example 3′ UTR is detected since the bar of the target RNA and for background binding to the MS2 loops only is comparable. In contrast, enrichment on the target RNA above the background is observed for miR-181b and miR-27a

low yields, it might be better to split the constructs into two or more parts.

3. XhoI and ApaI were used to insert the two MS2 stem-loop sequences into the pcDNA3.1(+) vector. Thus, cloning of the target sequence of interest with XhoI directly fuses the target with the MS2 loops without preventing having extra nucleotides between the two sequences.
4. The two MS2 loops alone serve as background control in the miRNA enrichment assay. MiRNAs binding to the MS2 loops will be excluded from the candidate list and not used for further validation.
5. RNA larger than 500 nt can barely be resolved using denaturing polyacrylamide (PAA) gel electrophoresis [23]. Therefore, denaturing agarose gel electrophoresis is used for constructs larger than 500 nt and sufficient to estimate the success of the transcription reaction and to check for RNA integrity. 1% agarose gels are run for 15 min at 80 V in 1× TAE. Bands are visualized under UV light due to addition of ethidium bromide to the gel solution.
6. 10^6 cells are sufficient for one target RNA + one MS2 control + 1 beads control + 1 input preparation. If more than one target RNA will be at a time, the number of cells needs to increase by 2.5×10^6/reaction.

7. The extract should be always prepared on the same day of the miRNA enrichment procedure and used fresh without freezing and thawing.
8. Ampicillin is the selection pressure for the pMalC_MS2BP-MBP pDNA, and chloramphenicol serves as selection pressure for the strain.
9. IPTG removes the transcriptional repressor from the promoter of the T7 RNA polymerase, which is endogenously introduced into the DE3 strain. Since the pMalC plasmid contains a T7 promoter, the MS2BP-MBP mRNA is produced and translated into protein by *E. coli* BL21(DE3)pLysS cells upon IPTG addition.
10. Preparation of pellet sample for gel run: use tip to take a little bit of the pellet, and resuspend it briefly in 500 μL 1 M Tris–HCl/6 M urea in 1.5 mL tube.
    (a) 3 μL pellet + 12 μL 1 M Tris–HCl/6 M Urea + 5 μL SDS load → load 20 μL
    (b) 3 μL supernatant + 12 μL 1 M Tris–HCl/6 M Urea + 5 μL SDS load → load 20 μL
11. Amylose resin binds 6–8 mg of MBP/mL bed.
12. Do not let the resin dry out! Close the column after the wash step, and keep it moisturized until further use.
13. Fractions with high sugar content tend to precipitate upon denaturation. It does not interfere with gel run, nevertheless elution fractions should be diluted at least 1:5 with water to prevent precipitation.
14. It is optimal to remove as much ethanol or buffer as possible. Therefore, the use of a needle under vacuum pressure at the end of the washing steps is recommended.
15. The rotation speed of the samples on the turning wheel should not be too fast otherwise the solution remains on the bottom of the tube due to centrifugal force. An optimal speed for the device used in the protocol here is 30 rpm.
16. BSA and yeast tRNA are added for blocking the beads' surface, which is not covered by the MS2BP-MBP protein to prevent unspecific binding of cell extract components to the beads.
17. If the required volume of the RNA samples is less than 10 μL, it is recommended to add nuclease-free H_2O to the RNA samples in order to avoid any loss. Glycogen might interfere with downstream applications like RNA-seq.
18. Since the two MS2 loop RNA is mostly much shorter than the target RNAs, the binding efficiency is consequently higher. An approximate 5× better immobilization rate was determined for the two MS2 loops in comparison to the example target RNA

used in the protocol. Therefore, the amount of the two MS2 loop RNA was adjusted to 5× less pmol to ensure similar amounts of RNA on the beads. It is recommended to test the binding efficiency of every target RNA and the two MS2 RNA only in order to determine a suitable ratio for immobilization.

19. A typical mixture of phenol and chloroform is 5:1 and 1:1 (v/v). At acidic pH, a 5:1 ratio results in the absence of DNA from the upper aqueous phase; whereas a 1:1 ratio provides maximal recovery of all RNAs but also results in maintaining some DNA present in the upper aqueous phase. Isoamyl alcohol is often added to prevent foaming (typically in a ratio of 24 parts chloroform to 1 part isoamyl alcohol) [24].
20. RNA can be precipitated by adding 1 volume of isopropanol or 2.5 volumes of ethanol and mixing thoroughly.
21. Kits for first-strand cDNA synthesis of miRNAs are available, usually based on reverse transcribing miRNAs after their artificial polyadenylation.
22. As an alternative to SYBR green-based qRT-PCR, TaqMan probes have shown to increase specificity and sensitivity for quantifying miRNAs. A detailed protocol is presented in ref. 21.

References

1. Hanahan D, Weinberg RA (2011) Hallmarks of cancer: the next generation. Cell 144 (5):646–674. https://doi.org/10.1016/j.cell.2011.02.013
2. Eichmüller SB, Osen W, Mandelboim O et al (2017) Immune modulatory microRNAs involved in tumor attack and tumor immune escape. J Natl Cancer Inst 109(10). https://doi.org/10.1093/jnci/djx034
3. Seliger B (2017) Immune modulatory microRNAs as a novel mechanism to revert immune escape of tumors. Cytokine Growth Factor Rev 36:49–56. https://doi.org/10.1016/j.cytogfr.2017.07.001
4. Braun J, Misiak D, Busch B et al (2014) Rapid identification of regulatory microRNAs by miTRAP (miRNA trapping by RNA in vitro affinity purification). Nucleic Acids Res 42(8): e66. https://doi.org/10.1093/nar/gku127
5. Gao F, Zhao Z, Zhao W et al (2013) miR-9 modulates the expression of interferon-regulated genes and MHC class I molecules in human nasopharyngeal carcinoma cells. Biochem Biophys Res Commun 431 (3):610–616. https://doi.org/10.1016/j.bbrc.2012.12.097
6. Wang B, Wang Q, Wang Z et al (2014) Metastatic consequences of immune escape from NK cell cytotoxicity by human breast cancer stem cells. Cancer Res 74(20):5746–5757. https://doi.org/10.1158/0008-5472.CAN-13-2563
7. Xie J, Liu M, Li Y et al (2014) Ovarian tumor-associated microRNA-20a decreases natural killer cell cytotoxicity by downregulating MICA/B expression. Cell Mol Immunol 11 (5):495–502. https://doi.org/10.1038/cmi.2014.30
8. Wang X, Li J, Dong K et al (2015) Tumor suppressor miR-34a targets PD-L1 and functions as a potential immunotherapeutic target in acute myeloid leukemia. Cell Signal 27 (3):443–452. https://doi.org/10.1016/j.cellsig.2014.12.003
9. Kulkarni S, Qi Y, O'hUigin C et al (2013) Genetic interplay between HLA-C and MIR148A in HIV control and Crohn disease. Proc Natl Acad Sci U S A 110 (51):20705–20710. https://doi.org/10.1073/pnas.1312237110
10. Jasinski-Bergner S, Stoehr C, Bukur J et al (2015) Clinical relevance of miR-mediated

HLA-G regulation and the associated immune cell infiltration in renal cell carcinoma. Oncoimmunology 4(6):e1008805. https://doi.org/10.1080/2162402X.2015.1008805
11. Cheng Z, Ma R, Tan W et al (2014) MiR-152 suppresses the proliferation and invasion of NSCLC cells by inhibiting FGF2. Exp Mol Med 46:e112. https://doi.org/10.1038/emm.2014.51
12. Chen L, Gibbons DL, Goswami S et al (2014) Metastasis is regulated via microRNA-200/ZEB1 axis control of tumour cell PD-L1 expression and intratumoral immunosuppression. Nat Commun 5:5241. https://doi.org/10.1038/ncomms6241
13. Johansson HE, Liljas L, Uhlenbeck OC (1997) RNA recognition by the MS2 phage coat protein. Semin Virol 8(3):176–185. https://doi.org/10.1006/smvy.1997.0120
14. Chamberlin M, Ring J (1973) Characterization of T7-specific ribonucleic acid polymerase. 1. General properties of the enzymatic reaction and the template specificity of the enzyme. J Biol Chem 248(6):2235–2244
15. Jurica MS, Licklider LJ, Gygi SR et al (2002) Purification and characterization of native spliceosomes suitable for three-dimensional structural analysis. RNA 8(4):426–439
16. Schneider CA, Rasband WS, Eliceiri KW (2012) NIH image to ImageJ: 25 years of image analysis. Nat Methods 9(7):671–675
17. Wang D, Zhang Z, O'Loughlin E et al (2012) Quantitative functions of Argonaute proteins in mammalian development. Genes Dev 26 (7):693–704. https://doi.org/10.1101/gad.182758.111
18. Agarwal V, Bell GW, Nam J et al (2015) Predicting effective microRNA target sites in mammalian mRNAs. Elife 4. https://doi.org/10.7554/eLife.05005
19. Kertesz M, Iovino N, Unnerstall U et al (2007) The role of site accessibility in microRNA target recognition. Nat Genet 39 (10):1278–1284. https://doi.org/10.1038/ng2135
20. Betel D, Koppal A, Agius P et al (2010) Comprehensive modeling of microRNA targets predicts functional non-conserved and non-canonical sites. Genome Biol 11(8):R90. https://doi.org/10.1186/gb-2010-11-8-r90
21. Kramer MF (2011) Stem-loop RT-qPCR for miRNAs. Curr Protoc Mol Biol Chapter 15: Unit 15.10. https://doi.org/10.1002/0471142727.mb1510s95
22. Chen C, Ridzon DA, Broomer AJ et al (2005) Real-time quantification of microRNAs by stem-loop RT-PCR. Nucleic Acids Res 33 (20):e179. https://doi.org/10.1093/nar/gni178
23. Summer H, Grämer R, Dröge P (2009) Denaturing urea polyacrylamide gel electrophoresis (urea PAGE). J Vis Exp 32:1485. https://doi.org/10.3791/1485
24. Kedzierski W, Porter JC (1991) A novel non-enzymatic procedure for removing DNA template from RNA transcription mixtures. Biotechniques 10(2):210–214

Part II

Functional Assays

Chapter 7

Expansion of Tumor-Infiltrating Lymphocytes from Melanoma Tumors

Stina Wickström and Tanja Lövgren

Abstract

Autologous, in vitro-expanded tumor-infiltrating lymphocytes (TIL) have been successfully used for treatment of melanoma patients. Expansion of TIL from tumors is usually performed in two steps. The details of the procedure differ between different laboratories, but the general concept remains the same. In the first step, small fragments of a tumor are placed in culture medium containing one or more T cell stimulating growth factors. Here the most common protocol using interleukin (IL)-2 is described. The length of the first step is flexible to allow generation of enough cell to start the second step of the procedure. The second step is a so-called rapid expansion protocol (REP) where harvested TIL from the first step are induced to massive proliferation via triggering of their T cell receptor (TCR) complex in presence of an excess of feeder cells and, again, T cell stimulating growth factors. This second expansion step is usually around 2 weeks in length. Here will be described a REP that uses soluble anti-CD3 antibodies for TCR triggering, irradiated peripheral blood mononuclear cells (PBMC) as feeder cells, and IL-2 as the T cell growth factor. Furthermore, the described protocol utilizes gas-permeable cell culture flasks that yield large number of cells similar to conventional bioreactors but using standard laboratory equipment.

Key words Immunotherapy, T cells, Tumor-infiltrating lymphocytes, In vitro expansion, Adoptive cell transfer, Interleukine-2, Anti-CD3, Feeder cells, Gas-permeable cell culture flasks

1 Introduction

Treatment of melanoma patients by adoptive transfer of autologous, in vitro expanded tumor-infiltrating lymphocytes (TIL) has shown impressive clinical results. The TIL adoptive cell therapy (ACT) field was pioneered by the research group of Professor Steven Rosenberg at the National Cancer Institute (NCI), and the first reports of successful TIL ACT in melanoma patients were published already in 1988 [1, 2]. Thereafter many other groups have performed TIL ACT trials in melanoma with similar success rate [3–9].

The efficacy of TIL ACT therapy in melanoma has been shown to depend on several factors. First, there is a need to precondition the patient with immunosuppressive chemotherapy. Without this

Yago Pico de Coaña (ed.), *Immune Checkpoint Blockade: Methods and Protocols*, Methods in Molecular Biology, vol. 1913, https://doi.org/10.1007/978-1-4939-8979-9_7, © Springer Science+Business Media, LLC, part of Springer Nature 2019

preconditioning, the TIL will not persist and the treatment will in most cases be unsuccessful. The preconditioning is thought to eradicate immunosuppressive immune cells and in parallel create a niche for the infused TIL with increased availability of stimulatory soluble factors and cell–cell interactions after deletion of competing T cells. Second, the infused TIL are often supported by infusions of IL-2 or other cytokines that support T cell survival and expansion.

Third, and in relation to the protocol presented here, the characteristics of the infused TIL product have a strong influence on the outcome of the treatment. Infusion of higher number of cells is generally correlated to better treatment outcome [4, 9]. However, the quality of the cell product does also play a role, and so-called young TIL cultured for a shorter time are superior to TIL cultured longer.

Most laboratories have their own protocol for stimulating the outgrowth and expansion of TIL from tumors. However, all protocols are derived from the protocols of the Rosenberg group, and the general procedures are the same. The TIL expansion is usually divided into two parts (Fig. 1). First, a resected tumor or a tumor biopsy is divided into small fragments (or even single-cell suspensions) that are placed into cell culture medium with T cell stimulating growth factors. Once enough TIL numbers are achieved, which usually takes between 2 and 4 weeks, they are subjected to a rapid expansion protocol (REP) where proliferation is stimulated by triggering of the T cell receptor complex in presence of T cell stimulating growth factors and feeder cells. The feeder cells are added to the cultures in excess, using 100–300-fold more feeder cells than added TIL. The amount of TIL in the starting culture is low, usually in the range of 1×10^3–1×10^4 TIL per ml cell culture medium. The REP cultures are usually harvested after around 2 weeks and will then yield up to several 1000-fold more TIL than was added at the REP start.

The current protocol will describe expanding TIL from melanoma tumors by first culturing tumor fragments in 24-well culture plates in presence of high-dose IL-2. After 2–4-week expansion, the cells are harvested and subjected to a REP. To start the REP, a small amount of TIL is added to gas-permeable culture flasks [10–13] with an excess of irradiated autologous or allogeneic PBMC as feeder cells, in presence of anti-CD3 antibodies and high-dose IL-2. The medium used throughout the protocol is vended as serum-free but is still supplemented with 2% autologous or allogeneic human serum since this dramatically increases T cell expansion. In summary, the protocol to expand TIL from tumors is straightforward. However, there are many hands-on tips and tricks that will facilitate the procedure and improve both the quantity and quality of the generated cells.

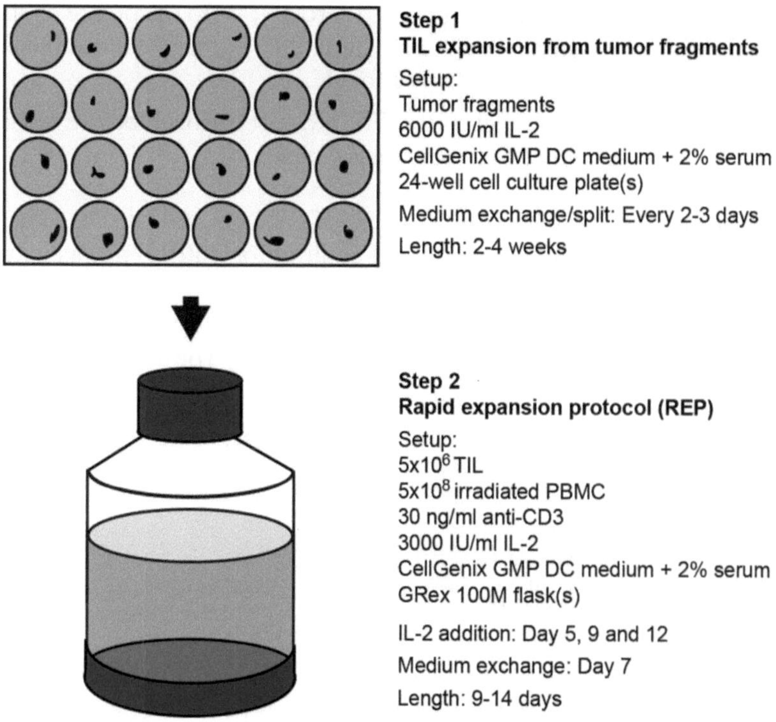

Fig. 1 General work scheme for expanding tumor-infiltrating lymphocytes (TIL) from melanoma tumors. The procedure is divided into two steps. Step 1 for expanding TIL from tumor material and step 2 for massively increasing the amount of TIL obtained in the first step by a rapid expansion (REP) protocol

2 Materials

2.1 General

1. General cell culture equipment and plastics such as pipettes, tips, tubes, etc.
2. LAF-bench.
3. Cell culture incubator set at 37C, 5% CO_2.
4. Centrifuge with swing-out rotor.
5. Microscope.
6. Inverted microscope.
7. Cell counter or counting chamber for manual counting.
8. 0.4% Trypan blue.
9. Complete cell culture medium: CellGenix GMP DC medium (CellGenix, *see* **Note 1**) supplemented with 2% human serum (autologous or a mix of allogeneic donor AB-serum, *see* **Note 2**).
10. IL-2 (*see* **Note 3**).

11. Optional: If the TIL product is frozen before starting the REP step. Freezing medium. 90% human serum supplemented with 10% dimethyl sulfoxide.
12. Optional: If the TIL product is frozen before starting the REP step. Cell freezing container.

2.2 Expansion of TIL from Tumor Material

1. Transport medium. CellGenix GMP DC medium (CellGenix) + optional addition of 100 U/ml penicillin/100 μg/ml streptomycin.
2. Initial culture medium. Complete cell culture medium + optional addition of 100 U/ml penicillin/100 μg/ml streptomycin.
3. Transport vessel. Sterile vessel with appropriate size for the resected tumor/biopsy.
4. Petri dishes.
5. Sterile tweezers.
6. Scalpels.
7. 24-well cell culture plates (*see* **Note 4**).

2.3 Rapid Expansion Protocol

1. Water bath set at 37 °C.
2. G-Rex 100 M gas-permeable flasks (Wilson Wolf, *see* **Note 4**).
3. OKT3, anti-CD3 antibody (*see* **Note 5**).
4. PBMC (autologous or a mix of PBMC from allogeneic blood donors, *see* **Note 2**).
5. Optional: Thawing medium for TIL in case the TIL product from the first expansion step was frozen. 9 mg/ml NaCl supplemented with 8% anticoagulant citrate dextrose solution.
6. Optional: If feeder cells are of lower or unknown quality (*see* **Note 6**). Pulmozyme buffer. 0.025 mg/ml Pulmozyme (Roche) and 2.5 mM $MgCl_2$ in cell culture medium.
7. Optional: In case the product is to be reinfused to a patient (*see* **Note 7**). Infusion buffer. 9 mg/ml NaCl supplemented with 2.5% human serum albumin (HSA).

3 Methods

3.1 Expansion of TIL from Tumor Material

1. The starting material for the TIL expansion is a resected tumor or a tumor biopsy (*see* **Note 8**). The tumor sample is transported to the laboratory in a sterile transport vessel in transport medium, consisting of cell culture medium with or without antibiotics (*see* **Note 9**).
2. 1.5 ml complete cell culture medium containing 6000 IU/ml IL-2 and with optional addition of antibiotics (*see* **Note 9**) is

added to wells of a 24-well plate. The number of wells that are prepared is adjusted depending on the amount of tumor material received.

3. The tumor is picked up from the transport vessel using sterile tweezers and placed in a petri dish. From this point, it is important work quickly to avoid that the tissue dries.
4. The tumor is cut free from as much surrounding tissue as possible. Especially important is to remove any skin still left since this is a large risk factor for microbial contaminations (*see* **Note 9**).
5. The tumor is cut into small fragments of approximately 1–3 mm^3, which are each placed into the wells that were previously prefilled with medium.
6. The plates are placed in a cell culture incubator.
7. One day after setup and thereafter every second to third day, the wells are monitored for contamination and TIL outgrowth by inspecting each well with an inverted microscope.
8. Contaminated wells (*see* **Note 9**). Wells contaminated with microbes are discarded. Contamination will usually result in medium color change and foggy cultures visible by eye, but in some cases, microbes grow slowly and will only be visible under the microscope. Work carefully to avoid infecting other wells. Empty infected wells. Handle suspicious wells as separate from other wells as possible, by changing all pipette tips etc. in between wells.
9. TIL-containing wells. TIL can be distinguished by their roundish to slightly elongated shape and their preference of growing in smaller or larger clusters. Wells where the bottom is covered to at least 50% with TIL are split into one more well by gently resuspending the content of the well by pipetting up and down with a 1 ml pipette tip and transferring half (or less) the volume to one or two new well. Fresh complete cell culture medium supplemented with 6000 IU/ml IL-2 is then added to each split well. The choice of splitting to one or more wells is made by taking into consideration the confluency of the well, the expansion rate of the cells, and the time to the next monitoring.
10. Remaining wells. For all wells that are not split, half of the medium is exchanged for new medium by carefully pipetting off 0.75 ml medium from the top of the well without disturbing the cells on the bottom and thereafter adding 0.75 ml fresh complete cell culture medium supplemented with 6000 IU/ml IL-2.
11. When it's estimated that enough TIL have grown out from the tumor to be able to start the REP, the cells are harvested (*see* **Note 10**). For each well where the bottom is completely

covered, there are around 1–2 × 10^6 of TIL. For each G-Rex 100 M flask that will be set up for the REP, 5 × 10^6 TIL are needed. Depending on the amount of tumor that was received, the efficacy of the TIL outgrowth and the number of G-Rex flasks to be set up, the first part of the TIL expansion usually takes between 2 and 4 weeks. The shorter side of the time range is preferable. Harvest the TIL by pipetting up and down with a 1 ml pipet tip. During the harvest, TIL from several wells are mixed to a bulk TIL product. Do not pool wells that contain no or very little TIL, wells with a lot of debris/cell death, or where contamination is suspected (*see* **Note 9**).

12. If REP is started from fresh TIL, make sure that all reagents for starting the REP, including thawing and irradiation of feeder cells, are ready before harvesting. Then harvest the cells as described above and in the REP section.
13. Optional: If REP cannot be started immediately, the TIL can be frozen (*see* **Note 11**). Harvest the cells as described above, count and determine viability by trypan blue staining, and thereafter centrifuge the tubes at 300 × *g* for 7 min. Add 1 ml freezing medium per 5–200 × 10^6 viable TIL depending on cell numbers needed further ahead. Distribute into cryotubes and place in a freezing container that is placed in a −80 °C freezer for at least 1 day before being transferred to a −150 °C freezer/liquid nitrogen.

3.2 Rapid Expansion Protocol

1. Optional: If TIL were frozen after the first expansion step, they should be thawed and rested for 1–2 days in complete cell culture medium with 6000 IU/ml IL-2 before REP is started.
2. Thawing is performed in a 37 °C water bath.
3. Thereafter the cells are quickly transferred to a tube with 10 ml thawing medium for TIL and are centrifuged at 300 × *g* for 7 min.
4. The cells are resuspended in complete cell culture medium supplemented with 6000 IU/ml IL-2 aiming to have more than 1 × 10^6 cells per ml.
5. The cells are counted and viability determined by trypan blue staining.
6. Concentration is adjusted to 1 × 10^6 viable TIL/ml with complete cell culture medium supplemented with 6000 IU/ml IL-2.
7. The cells are plated with 1.5 ml per well in a 24-well plate.
8. When the REP is to be started, the TIL are harvested as described in the section describing the first part of the expansion and below.

9. Each G-Rex 100 M flask is filled with 875 ml of complete cell culture medium with 3000 IU/ml IL-2 and placed in the cell culture incubator for warming the medium.
10. Prepare tubes for thawing feeder cells. One 50 ml tube filled with 40 ml complete cell culture medium, with or without the addition of Pulmozyme plus $MgCl_2$ (*see* **Note 6**), for up to 1.5×10^9 PBMC. 0.5×10^9 feeder cells are needed for each G-Rex 100 M flask, but thawing tends to result in losses of up to 50% of the cells. Thus, it is suggested to thaw up to the double amount of PBMC. The PBMC should either be autologous or a mix from at least three allogeneic donors that have been appropriately tested for viral infections (*see* **Note 2**).
11. Thawing is performed in a 37 °C water bath.
12. Thereafter the cells are quickly transferred to the prepared tubes.
13. The tubes are irradiated at 40 Gy.
14. The tubes are centrifuged at $300 \times g$ for 7 min.
15. The cells are resuspended in a few ml of complete medium (to avoid aggregates) and then filled up to 40 ml complete cell culture medium with 3000 IU/ml IL-2.
16. If there are visible aggregates, try to dissolve these by pipetting. If impossible, remove the aggregates with the pipette. Aggregates are sticky and can lead to decreased final TIL yields.
17. The cells are counted and viability is determined by trypan blue staining.
18. For each G-Rex flask to be set up, 100 ml of cell suspension containing in total 0.5×10^9 viable PBMC in complete cell culture medium with 3000 IU/ml IL-2 are prepared.
19. OKT3 antibody is added to the feeder mix to a concentration of 300 ng/ml (final concentration in the G-Rex 100 M flask is 30 ng/ml).
20. 100 ml of feeder/OKT3 mix is added to each G-Rex flask.
21. The TIL are harvested as described in the section covering the first part of the TIL expansion.
22. Count and determine viability by trypan blue staining.
23. Take off 5×10^6 TIL into a tube for each G-Rex flask to be set up. The rest can be frozen as described in the first part of the TIL expansion (unless the REP is started from previously frozen TIL, which should not be refrozen).
24. Centrifuge at $300 \times g$ for 7 min.
25. Resuspend with 25 ml complete cell culture medium supplemented with 3000 IU/ml IL-2 per 5×10^6 cells.
26. 25 ml TIL suspension is added to each G-Rex 100 M flask.

27. The flasks are placed in a cell culture incubator.
28. On day 5, new IL-2 is added to the flasks to a final concentration of 3000 IU/ml (making the assumption that all IL-2 has been consumed).
29. On day 7, the medium is refreshed. Half, i.e., 500 ml, of conditioned medium is carefully pipetted off the flasks without disturbing the cells on the bottom, and 500 ml fresh complete cell culture medium containing 6000 IU/ml IL-2 is added (final concentration 3000 IU/ml, making the assumption that all IL-2 has been consumed).
30. On day 9, new IL-2 is added to the flasks to a final concentration of 3000 IU/ml (making the assumption that all IL-2 has been consumed). From day 9, one can also choose to harvest the cells. This will yield somewhat fewer but possibly less exhausted cells.
31. On day 12, new IL-2 is added to the flasks to a final concentration of 3000 IU/ml (making the assumption that all IL-2 has been consumed).
32. Latest on day 14, the cells are harvested. In general, each G-Rex will at this point yield 2–5 $\times$ 10^9 TIL.
33. Pipette off and discard as much medium as possible without disturbing the cells on the bottom of the flasks. Generally, at least 700 ml can be discarded.
34. Resuspend cells by agitating the flasks with a rotating movement.
35. Harvest the cells into centrifuge tubes.
36. Count and determine viability by trypan blue staining.
37. Centrifuge at 300 $\times$ *g* for 7 min.
38. If the cells are to be infused into the patient (*see* **Note 7**), they are resuspended in infusion buffer and centrifuged again at 300 $\times$ *g* for 7 min. The supernatant is discarded, and the cell pellet is resuspended in infusion buffer and transferred to an infusion bag. More infusion buffer is added to the bag until the cell concentration is 20–150 $\times$ 10^6 per ml.
39. If the cells are to be frozen, they are resuspended in freezing medium, 1 ml per 20–200 $\times$ 10^6 cells, and distributed in cryovials. Place in a freezing container that is placed in a −80 °C freezer for at least 1 day before being transferred to a −150 °C freezer/liquid nitrogen.

4 Notes

1. The protocol describes using CellGenix GMP DC medium (CellGenix) + 2% human serum throughout both the

expansion steps. This serum-free medium is a GMP grade medium optimized for DC generation but does also work for T cell expansion. However, for efficient T cell expansion, it should be supplemented with 2% human serum. This medium can be exchanged to another medium suitable for culturing T cells, but if another serum-free medium is chosen, the cell yields will in most cases be improved by adding serum especially during the early parts of the protocol. Some protocols switch culture medium during the TIL expansion, usually to move from a higher serum content in the beginning to serum-free medium in the end of the expansion.

2. There is a reduced risk to use autologous serum and feeder cellsfor the TIL expansion, with no possibility for donor-derived infections or immune reactions. However, there are some disadvantages. It is often hard to get enough serum and feeders from the patient. There is also a risk that autologous blood products are immunosuppressive, due to the cancer. In addition, the alloreaction between the TIL and allogeneic feeders is thought to enhance the expansion. Thus, although autologous feeders and plasma has been used [8], most laboratories use allogeneicproducts. However, these products obviously have to be confirmed safe by microbial testing. Regarding the serum, only male AB-serum should be used. As for the feeders, mixed irradiated PBMC from three or more allogeneic blood donors are usually used. Several donors should be mixed to dilute the risk that one has a negative impact on the TIL expansion, but to ensure good results, the feeders should be pretested for ability to expand T cells. In addition, to make sure that no viable feeder cellsare present at the day of TIL harvest, feeder-only cultures (containing irradiated PBMC, anti-CD3, and IL-2but no TIL) should be set up in parallel to the REP.

3. During both the initial stimulation of TIL outgrowth from tumor fragments and the REP, T cell stimulating growth factor(s) are added. The most common is IL-2, but also here other cytokines have been used and suggested to result in a better quality TIL product. For example, IL-7, IL-15, or IL-21 stimulated T cell expansion has been reported to result in more memory and/or stem cell like T cell subsets [14–18].

4. There are also different cell culture vessels used. In the first expansion step, most groups use plates, but also larger culture vessels may be used. The advantage of using plates is that TIL do not grow out from all fragments, and with plates one has the opportunity to choose the wells where TIL are growing. In addition, if infection/contamination occurs, it could be limited to some of the wells, and the rest of the wells can be rescued instead of discarding the whole TIL culture. Further, one can

also test the different wells for functionality, although this is seldom done since it adds more time to the culture protocol.

In the REP, cultures are usually set up in static flasks, and fresh medium is added, or cultures are split as the expansion proceeds. The static cultures may be kept throughout the expansion, but the cell yield is markedly increased by moving the culture into bioreactors after a couple of days, which allows for continuous control of medium condition and cell concentration [21, 22]. However, bioreactors are not standard equipment in most laboratories, and, in addition, using them increases the consumption of medium and thereby the costs massively. An alternative to bioreactors are the gas-permeable G-Rex flasks that are used in the described protocol [10–13]. These are static but have a large gas-permeable membrane in the bottom, where the cells will sediment. Since the gas exchange takes place in the bottom of the flasks, they can be filled with more medium than standard flasks, minimizing the need for manipulation. The flasks are placed in a normal cell incubator and may therefore be used in any standard laboratory. Medium exchange can be performed manually, although there are also closed system variantsof the flasks with tubing which can be connected to a medium pump.

5. During the REP the TIL expansion is stimulated by triggering the TCR complex. In the described protocol, only the CD3 is targeted by agonisticantibodies, but there are publications that suggest that a combined triggering of the TCR complex and costimulatory molecules such as CD28 or 4-1BB may result in a superior TIL product [14, 18–20]. Furthermore, some protocols use agonistic antibodies immobilized on culture vessel surfaces, onto microbeads, or on artificial APC. Still, the most used variant is to trigger the TCR via soluble anti-CD3 antibodies as in the described protocol. However, even though the anti-CD3 is in this case simply added to the cultures, the idea is that they are bound via Fc receptors to feeder cellsthat are added in excess into the culture.

6. The quality of the feeder cells is essential for the expansion in the REP. The protocol here describes adding 100-fold more feeder cells than TIL, and using a lower feeder cell to TIL ratio will result in lower yields. Thus, there is a need for large numbers of feeder cells.

One problem that may arise is the formation of cell aggregates in the PBMCused as feeder cells during thawingand/or irradiation. Presence of aggregates will lead to that the feeder cells are less available and will reflect using a too low number of feeder cells. In addition, aggregates are sticky and may also stick to TIL cells, leading to a lower final yield.
The formation of cell aggregates in the feeders may be due to contamination of the PBMC with thrombocytes and/or

granulocytes or presence of dead cells. Cell aggregation can be avoided by carefully following the standard protocol for PBMC preparation, including a slow speed centrifugation to decrease thrombocyte frequency. If a leukapheresis product is instead used as the source for PBMC, the leukapheresis should be set up with the goal to limit the amount of granulocytes in the product. In addition, correctly performed freezingand thawingis important to avoid high frequencies of dead cells in the thawed PBMC, which is always associated with aggregate formation. In addition, the optional Pulmozyme and $MgCl_2$ buffer can be used independently of feeder origin to minimize the risk of aggregates when thawingand irradiationof the feeder cells. Finally, if aggregates anyway appear in the PBMC, attempts to dissolve the clumps should be done, and if not successful, the clumps should be removed.

7. If the cell product is to be used for actual patient therapy, the work has to be performed in compliance with good manufacturing practice (GMP), in clean room facilities, and all materials have to be certified accordingly. Sterility testing should be performed at different time points during the procedure, following local regulations.
8. Tumors may be from the skin, lymph nodes, or other organs. The tumor location may play a role for the outcome. For example, skin may be contaminated with microbes, while lymph node metastases may contain more irrelevant T cells, and tumor material from different organs may contain other cells such as fibroblasts that may take over the culture.

   One can use either large resected tumors or small biopsies. However, with less material, there is of course a risk that the expansion will take longer time which will decrease the quality of the TIL product.

   Some research groups use enzymatic digestion or mechanical disassociation of the tumor to produce a single-cell suspensionthat is used as starting material for the TIL outgrowth. This method can certainly work as well as plating small fragments. However, it does make monitoring more difficult, and there is, for example, harder to see when a well should be split and also a greater risk that microbial contaminations are missed.
9. Tumor material resected by operation may be contaminated from the beginning by commensal or pathogenic microbes from the patient or become contaminated through the operation procedures. To limit the risks for contamination, the material may, as described above, be transported and cultures set up in medium containing antibiotics in order to eradicate any contaminating bacteria. However, using antibiotics throughout the culture may instead hide smoldering infections and is therefore advised against.

Dissecting out the actual tumor material will also limit the risk of microbial contamination. In particular, traces of the skin should be carefully removed. Furthermore, if several tumor samples are received, these should as much as possible be handled separately. However, most importantly is careful monitoring of every well at frequent intervals and separately handling wells suspected to be contaminated at an early stage. Note that some infections will only be visible under the microscopeand may grow very slowly.

10. The first step, where TIL are expanded from tumor fragments is flexible in length. This is necessary as the amount of tumor material received will differ between patients. In addition, outgrowth of TIL may in some cases be slow, possibly due to low numbers of TIL being present in the tumor or TIL being compromised by exhaustion or suppressive mechanisms inside the tumor. Since there is such a clear connection between the number of cells infused and the treatment efficacy, it is tempting to simply culture the cells for longer to be able to start more G-Rex 100 M flasks in the REP. However, too long culture risks generating exhausted and/or terminally differentiated cells and the cells should preferentially be cultured no more than 3 weeks. Thus, balancing cell numbers and culture time is one of the difficulties of the TIL expansion protocol, and this can only be handled by notoriously caring for the TIL cultures. Culture time will be minimized by carefully monitoring the wells, splitting when needed and refreshing the medium regularly every 2–3 days, even if it does not look conditioned.

    It is possible to do prescreening of the TIL-containing wells for functionality, usually by analyzing recognition of tumor cells in vitro. However, any functionality testing does add to the time required for the expansion, and tumor cells have to be available for the testing. Therefore, most use unscreened TIL to start the REP protocol.

11. In addition to slow outgrowth of TIL, sometimes logistical issues may mean that the REP start is delayed. Then there is an option to freeze the expanded TIL, and thaw 1–2 days before the REP is to be started. However, freezingdoes have a negative impact on the TIL which also has to be weighted into the decision. If the delay is less than a week, freezing is probably a worse choice. There is also an option to freeze the final product, but it is advised to, if possible, avoid freezing and give the cell product fresh to the patient.

References

1. Rosenberg SA, Packard BS, Aebersold PM et al (1988) Use of tumor-infiltrating lymphocytes and interleukin-2 in the immunotherapy of patients with metastatic melanoma. A preliminary report. N Engl J Med 319 (25):1676–1680. https://doi.org/10.1056/NEJM198812223192527
2. Rosenberg SA, Yannelli JR, Yang JC et al (1994) Treatment of patients with metastatic melanoma with autologous tumor-infiltrating lymphocytes and interleukin 2. J Natl Cancer Inst 86(15):1159–1166
3. Besser MJ, Shapira-Frommer R, Schachter J (2015) Tumor-infiltrating lymphocytes: clinical experience. Cancer J 21(6):465–469. https://doi.org/10.1097/PPO.0000000000000154
4. Besser MJ, Shapira-Frommer R, Treves AJ et al (2010) Clinical responses in a phase II study using adoptive transfer of short-term cultured tumor infiltration lymphocytes in metastatic melanoma patients. Clin Cancer Res 16 (9):2646–2655. https://doi.org/10.1158/1078-0432.CCR-10-0041
5. Ellebaek E, Iversen TZ, Junker N et al (2012) Adoptive cell therapy with autologous tumor infiltrating lymphocytes and low-dose Interleukin-2 in metastatic melanoma patients. J Transl Med 10:169. https://doi.org/10.1186/1479-5876-10-169
6. Hinrichs CS, Rosenberg SA (2014) Exploiting the curative potential of adoptive T-cell therapy for cancer. Immunol Rev 257(1):56–71. https://doi.org/10.1111/imr.12132
7. Pilon-Thomas S, Kuhn L, Ellwanger S et al (2012) Efficacy of adoptive cell transfer of tumor-infiltrating lymphocytes after lymphopenia induction for metastatic melanoma. J Immunother 35(8):615–620. https://doi.org/10.1097/CJI.0b013e31826e8f5f
8. Poschke I, Lövgren T, Adamson L et al (2014) A phase I clinical trial combining dendritic cell vaccination with adoptive T cell transfer in patients with stage IV melanoma. Cancer Immunol Immunother 63(10):1061–1071. https://doi.org/10.1007/s00262-014-1575-2
9. Radvanyi LG, Bernatchez C, Zhang M et al (2012) Specific lymphocyte subsets predict response to adoptive cell therapy using expanded autologous tumor-infiltrating lymphocytes in metastatic melanoma patients. Clin Cancer Res 18(24):6758–6770. https://doi.org/10.1158/1078-0432.CCR-12-1177
10. Bajgain P, Mucharla R, Wilson J et al (2014) Optimizing the production of suspension cells using the G-Rex "M" series. Mol Ther Methods Clin Dev 1:14015. https://doi.org/10.1038/mtm.2014.15
11. Forget MA, Haymaker C, Dennison JB et al (2016) The beneficial effects of a gas-permeable flask for expansion of Tumor-Infiltrating lymphocytes as reflected in their mitochondrial function and respiration capacity. Oncoimmunology 5(2):e1057386. https://doi.org/10.1080/2162402X.2015.1057386
12. Forget MA, Malu S, Liu H et al (2014) Activation and propagation of tumor-infiltrating lymphocytes on clinical-grade designer artificial antigen-presenting cells for adoptive immunotherapy of melanoma. J Immunother 37 (9):448–460. https://doi.org/10.1097/CJI.0000000000000056
13. Jin J, Sabatino M, Somerville R et al (2012) Simplified method of the growth of human tumor infiltrating lymphocytes in gas-permeable flasks to numbers needed for patient treatment. J Immunother 35 (3):283–292. https://doi.org/10.1097/CJI.0b013e31824e801f
14. Alvarez-Fernandez C, Escriba-Garcia L, Vidal S et al (2016) A short CD3/CD28 costimulation combined with IL-21 enhance the generation of human memory stem T cells for adoptive immunotherapy. J Transl Med 14 (1):214. https://doi.org/10.1186/s12967-016-0973-y
15. Cieri N, Camisa B, Cocchiarella F et al (2013) IL-7 and IL-15 instruct the generation of human memory stem T cells from naive precursors. Blood 121(4):573–584. https://doi.org/10.1182/blood-2012-05-431718
16. Klebanoff CA, Finkelstein SE, Surman DR et al (2004) IL-15 enhances the in vivo antitumor activity of tumor-reactive CD8+ T cells. Proc Natl Acad Sci U S A 101(7):1969–1974. https://doi.org/10.1073/pnas.0307298101
17. Li Y, Bleakley M, Yee C (2005) IL-21 influences the frequency, phenotype, and affinity of the antigen-specific CD8 T cell response. J Immunol 175(4):2261–2269
18. Redeker A, Arens R (2016) Improving adoptive T Cell therapy: the particular role of T cell costimulation, cytokines, and post-transfer vaccination. Front Immunol 7:345. https://doi.org/10.3389/fimmu.2016.00345
19. Chacon JA, Pilon-Thomas S, Sarnaik AA et al (2013) Continuous 4-1BB co-stimulatory signals for the optimal expansion of tumor-infiltrating lymphocytes for adoptive T-cell therapy. Oncoimmunology 2(9):e25581. https://doi.org/10.4161/onci.25581

20. Chacon JA, Wu RC, Sukhumalchandra P et al (2013) Co-stimulation through 4-1BB/CD137 improves the expansion and function of CD8(+) melanoma tumor-infiltrating lymphocytes for adoptive T-cell therapy. PLoS One 8(4):e60031. https://doi.org/10.1371/journal.pone.0060031
21. Donia M, Larsen SM, Met O et al (2014) Simplified protocol for clinical-grade tumor-infiltrating lymphocyte manufacturing with use of the Wave bioreactor. Cytotherapy 16(8):1117–1120. https://doi.org/10.1016/j.jcyt.2014.02.004
22. Klapper JA, Thomasian AA, Smith DM et al (2009) Single-pass, closed-system rapid expansion of lymphocyte cultures for adoptive cell therapy. J Immunol Methods 345(1-2):90–99. https://doi.org/10.1016/j.jim.2009.04.009

Chapter 8

Establishment of Two Dimensional (2D) and Three-Dimensional (3D) Melanoma Primary Cultures as a Tool for In Vitro Drug Resistance Studies

Nataly Cruz Rodríguez, Johanna Lineros, Carol Stefany Rodríguez, Lina María Martínez, and Josefa Antonia Rodríguez

Abstract

Characteristics of melanoma cells have been deciphered by studies carried out in two dimensional cell cultures growing as adherent monolayers on the bottom of plastic flasks. Melanoma cells can be cultured with a considerable degree of success, and, depending on the further use of the cells obtained in the culture, methodologies have to be adjusted to obtain reliable results. Although there are many melanoma continuous cell lines, in vitro 2D and 3D melanoma primary cell culture may be a more useful model to investigate interactions between cancer cells and immune system, as well as the effect of cytotoxic treatments and personalized medicine in environments more similar to the physiological conditions.

Here, we described a protocol which employs many strategies to obtain primary 2D and 3D melanoma cultures as a model to study cell–cell and cell–microenvironment interactions that must be considered to properly design personalized cancer treatments, as well as for testing novel anticancer drugs and drug delivery vehicles.

Key words Melanoma, Primary cell culture, Two dimensional cell culture, Three-dimensional cell spheroids, Cancer model, Drug resistance

1 Introduction

Metastatic melanoma is a highly aggressive and drug-resistant form of skin cancer, which remains fatal, despite advances in therapies, because tumors develop resistance to new therapeutic alternatives.

Reliable human screening models must be designed to improve translation of findings from basic cellular research into clinical applications. Advances in cell culture techniques have allowed the development of new in vitro strategies useful to study cancer biology [1]; however, so far, there is no model available that mimics all aspects of human cancer in vivo, and thus, therapeutic response and acquisition of therapy or cell death resistance are difficult to predict. As most people work with finite or continuous cell lines growing in

Yago Pico de Coaña (ed.), *Immune Checkpoint Blockade: Methods and Protocols*, Methods in Molecular Biology, vol. 1913, https://doi.org/10.1007/978-1-4939-8979-9_8, © Springer Science+Business Media, LLC, part of Springer Nature 2019

two dimensional culture, both the cell composition of the culture and its gene expression profile must be evaluated to determine if cultured cells are mostly mature and differentiated quiescent cells or if they are precursor cells that can proliferate but can't differentiate without induction conditions. Primary two dimensional adherent cell culture (2D cell culture) is a simple, convenient, and low-cost technique useful to develop protein expression, cytotoxicity, cell migration, and invasion assays.

Although melanoma cell lines are useful to investigate basic aspects of this type of skin cancer, primary melanoma tumors and continuous cell lines exhibit many differences because of many factors that occur during cell culture including (1) selection of cell population and lack of tumor cell interactions with normal stroma and immune cells [2], (2) alterations in gene expression profiles due to long-term culture that allow cells to overcome crisis and start growing in continuous culture with higher tumorigenicity [3], and (3) lack of tumor microenvironment. In uveal melanoma, it has been demonstrated that during the cell line establishment, multiple passaging alters gene expression [2]. Furthermore, continuous cell lines are composed of a selected homogeneous cell population, while primary tumor culture contained diversity of cell populations that interact among them and are selected as the culture progresses.

In vivo melanoma models using human melanoma cell lines are used for preclinical testing of anticancer therapies and studies of molecular biological mechanisms. Tumor cells are transplanted in immunosuppressed or genetically engineered mice, for spontaneous melanoma generation. After establishment of xenograft–melanoma, cells interact with murine stroma allowing the investigation of growth characteristics and drug response on human melanoma cells in vivo. Other animals have also been used, such as zebrafish, which are more suitable for imaging and high-throughput studies.

Most studies in melanoma cell biology and therapeutic drug activity have been done with 2D culture assays, a useful model to elucidate the basic principles of tumor cell biology. Cells in this model grown as a monolayer on culture flasks have uniformly distributed access to the culture medium components as well as oxygen and drugs tested on them.

Generally, treatments that do not work in 2D culture do not work either in more complex models. For this reason, this model is appropriate to perform preliminary tests to determine drug effects before using more sophisticated preclinical models.

Although conventional 2D culture can be used to perform protein expression, cytotoxicity, migration, and adhesion assays, as tumor cells in vivo grow in a three-dimensional space interacting with the stroma (ECM, fibroblasts, endothelial and immune cells infiltrating the tumor), two dimensional cultures cannot imitate this heterogeneity in vitro. Melanoma cancer cells grown in 2D cultures can easily be killed by low doses of chemotherapeutic drugs or low doses of radiation, while in vivo their activity can be affected by different factors such as the poor access of tumor cells to nutrients and oxygen, the metabolic conversion of drugs within the cells, or the effect of patient's immune response.

In view of the above, three-dimensional cell culture (3D culture) has been shown to markedly impact cellular morphology and signaling providing an environment that resembles human malignant melanoma in vivo. If melanoma cells grow in a 3D culture, they provide a more complex preclinical drug testing system for human malignant melanoma, useful for develop in vitro test systems. It has been reported that some of the cells growing in 3D culture may become resistant to therapy, similarly to cancer cells in vivo [4]. Consequently, this model is more valid for testing and discovering new drugs for cancer therapies. In addition, cells growing in 3D are also a more realistic model for testing drug penetration on the inside of a micro-tissue [5], indicating that tumor architecture and microenvironment could influence the drug response against melanoma cells.

Several methodologies to develop tumor spheroids in 3D cultures have been reported as an excellent model used in cancer biology and toxicology study. Tumor spheroids mimic avascular in vivo tumors and present similar diffusional limitations to the mass transfer of oxygen, nutrients, and waste through cell–cell interactions and cell–extracellular matrix interactions [6]. In this regard, tumor spheroids, which are easy to obtain without specialized equipment, remain a very useful tool for design in vitro platforms that allow understanding of specific aspects of each tumor [7] and to develop appropriate test drug delivery systems in a more physiological relevant situation when compared to 2D monolayer cell cultures taking into account that this model considers the pathophysiological gradients of drugs in in vivo tumors, allowing the improvement of clinical outcomes in response to therapy for malignant melanoma [8].

Several spheroid-generation techniques have been described in literature that can generate uniform spheroids with a defined size and cell number such as liquid overlay, hanging drop culture, use of Matrigel, agar-coated plates, and more recently described use of hanging drop array plate [6]. After 15 days of incubation at 37 °C, in 10% of CO_2 (*see* **Note 1**), spheroids generated reach a final diameter of approximately 500 μm of diameter which resembles micro metastasis or intercapillary micro regions of solid tumors [9, 10]. These spheroids can be allowed to grow and co-develop with a skin scaffold for 20–30 days [8].

2 Materials

2.1 Plastic

1. Petri dishes, 9 cm.
2. Flasks of 25 cm^2 or 24-well plates.
3. Pipettes 5–10 ml.
4. 50 ml sterile centrifuge tubes.
5. Blood sample tubes with EDTA.
6. Vacutainer needles.
7. Tourniquet.
8. Scalpels.
9. 24-well plates.
10. Forceps.
11. Cryotubes, 1.5–2.0 ml.
12. 15 ml sterile conical tubes.

2.2 Reagents

1. Noble agar.
2. Ultrapure water (UPW).
3. Trypsin EDTA 1×.
4. Trypan Blue, 0.4%.

2.3 Media and Buffers

1. Collection medium: Dulbecco's modification of Eagle's basal medium (DMEM) + 200 U/ml penicillin, 200 μg/ml streptomycin, and 5 μg/ml amphotericin β (*see* **Note 2**).
2. Decontamination medium: DMEM with 10% FBS and twice as many as a normal concentration of penicillin/streptomycin/amphotericin β.
3. Initiation medium: DMEM supplemented with 15% FBS, 250 U/ml penicillin, 0.25 mg/ml streptomycin, and 0.0025 mg/ml of amphotericin β, enriched with 5 μg/ml of insulin. Just before plating the cells, add 5% PRP of total medium volume contained within the plate.
4. Wash buffer: Dulbecco's phosphate-buffered saline (DPBS) without calcium and magnesium.
5. Melanoma growth medium: DMEM supplemented with FBS at 10%, 100 U/ml penicillin, 100 μg/ml streptomycin, and 0.0025 mg/ml of amphotericin β, enriched with 5 μg/ml of insulin.
6. Platelet-rich plasma (PRP): 10 ml of patient's whole blood collected in tubes with sodium citrate were centrifuged for 6 min at 378 × *g* at room temperature without brake. Aspirate the plasma fraction corresponding to the upper third that is above the buffy coat, which is known as the platelet-rich plasma

fraction. Platelets in PRP were counted manually in the hemocytometer.

7. Freezing medium (DFM): 10% DMSO in 90% fetal bovine serum (FBS).

2.4 Solutions

1. Collagenase IV solution: 200–250 unites of collagenase IV per ml of DMEM. Add HEPES to a final concentration of 100 μM, 5% FBS, 20 μg/ml final of gentamicin, and 2.5 μg/ml insulin. Sterilize solution by filtration through a 0.22 μm filter.
2. 70% ethanol: Mix in 1 L bottle 700 ml absolute ethanol plus 300 ml H_2O. Keep at room temperature.
3. Dissection PBS: PBSA with 2.5 pg/ml Fungizone, 100 U/ml penicillin, and 100 pg/ml streptomycin.

2.5 Special Equipment

1. Laminar-flow hoods.
2. Cell counter (hemocytometer).
3. Centrifuges.
4. CO_2 incubators.
5. Inverted and optical microscopes.
6. Canes for six 1.5–2.0 ml cryotubes (for nitrogen freezer).

3 Methods

To establish primary 2D and 3D melanoma cultures, and maintenance of the growing cultures, basic protocols of cell culture can be designed to easily adapted to the growth of almost all tumor types. Whole blood and biopsy samples were obtained from patients with malignant invasive melanoma according to TNM Classification for Malignant Melanoma [11, 12]. Work with human biopsies requires the approval of the local ethical committee and the patient informed consent. These techniques must be applied in sterile conditions and should be carried out in a Class II biological safety cabinet.

3.1 Biopsy Collection

Specimen collection must be coordinated with the operating room or pathology, and 50 ml sample tubes, properly marked and containing 10 ml of collection medium, were provided.

1. Once the tumor is removed from the patient, prior to leaving the sterile area, a tumor sample is obtained and placed into the 50 ml falcon with 20 ml of collection medium and immediately transported to the laboratory at room temperature (*see* **Note 3**).
2. Before starting sample processing, data must be recorded, and assign a code for every sample to identify each culture obtained and to guarantee the confidentiality of the patient's data.

3.2 Biopsy Decontamination

Although most surgical samples are sterile, specimens such as the skin, melanomas, and gastrointestinal or genitourinary biopsies are easy to contaminate despite the washing and disinfection carried out before surgery and administration of a parenteral antibiotic prior to surgery.

1. Immerse biopsy in 70% ethanol for 30 s to 1 min (*see* **Note 4**).
2. Rinse biopsy twice in wash buffer to clean off ethanol.
3. Immerse biopsy in decontamination medium for 10 min at room temperature (*see* **Note 5**).

3.3 Establishing Melanoma 2D Cell Cultures by Enzymatic Disaggregation

The first step in initiating primary melanoma culture is to separate cells from each other and from extracellular matrix components while maintaining cell viability to later grow the resulting cell suspension in culture. Depending on strategies used for cellular disintegration, primary cell culture can be initiated after mechanical (cut, chop) or enzymatic (active proteases like collagenase, dispase, trypsin, elastase, etc.) treatments (Fig. 1) (*see* **Note 6**).

Unlike normal human melanocytes culture which requires growth factors such as hepatocyte growth factor (HGF) [13, 14], or endothelin 1 [15], among others, melanoma cells from advanced lesions don't require a selective combination of growth factors to proliferate in culture. However, we use some strategies to obtain growth factors to improve melanoma growth in vitro (*see* **Note 7**).

1. Remove adipose or necrotic tissue with a scalpel.
2. Mince the remaining tissue into small pieces of about 1 mm^2 or smaller with a surgical scalpel blade (*see* **Note 8**).

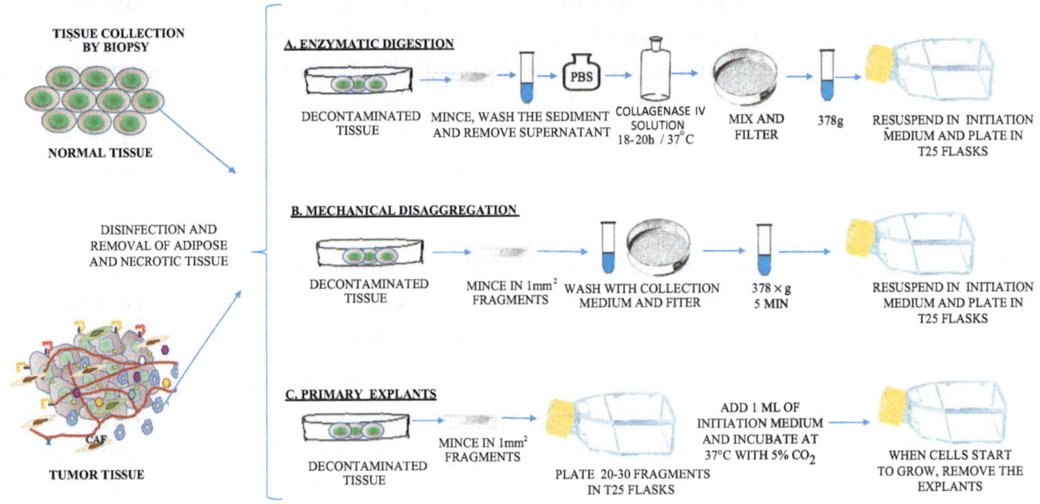

Fig. 1 Strategies used for disaggregation of cells to initiate primary culture in vitro

3. Disassociate melanoma cells from tissue by incubation in a collagenase IV solution for 18 to 20 h, at 37 °C (*see* **Note 9**).
4. Remove tissue from incubator and shake vigorously by pipetting up and down.
5. Filter the cell suspension through a series of sterile mesh with different pore sizes to remove clumps of partially digested tissue.
6. Centrifuge at 378 × *g* for 5 min at room temperature.
7. Discard supernatant and resuspend pellet in 5 ml of fresh medium.
8. Count cells in a hemocytometer.
9. Plate 1.5×10^5 cells per ml adding 5% PRP to initiating medium just before plating.
10. Seed the cellular suspension in 25 cm flasks and incubate in a humidified atmosphere at 37 °C and 10% CO_2.
11. After 24 h remove initiation medium and replace with melanoma growth medium enriched with PRP.
12. Examine cultures twice a week on inverted microscope to check the healthy status of the cells and cell density. Check also for normal fibroblastic growth, or piling up and random overgrowth, indicative of positive tumor cell growth.
13. Check for any sign of microbial contamination (*see* **Note 10**).
14. Change melanoma growth medium enriched with 5% PRP every 3 or 4 days until cells reach confluency.

3.4 Propagating Melanoma Culture

1. Once cells reach confluency, remove melanoma growth medium.
2. Wash cells with a half of the volume used to keep cells in culture.
3. Gently shake the culture flask to wash the cells and remove wash buffer (*see* **Note 11**).
4. Add 1 ml of trypsin EDTA 1×, and gently shake to distribute it over all the culture surface.
5. Incubate for 1–2 min at 37 °C (*see* **Note 12**).
6. Resuspend in the initial volume of fresh melanoma growth medium, and transfer cell suspension to a 15 ml centrifuge tube.
7. Centrifuge for 5 min at 378 × *g* and 4 °C.
8. Discard the supernatant and resuspend cells in 5 ml of fresh medium.
9. Count cells in triplicate and replate cells at $3–6 \times 10^4$ cells/ml.

3.5 Cell Counting

1. Trypsinize a monolayer culture as for routine subculture.
2. Resuspend cells diluting 50:50 with complete medium and mix well the cell suspension.
3. Clean the surface of the Neubauer chamber and the coverslip with 70% alcohol; put the coverslip over the counting area of the Neubauer chamber.
4. Mix the cell suspension and transfer 10 μl to a 1.5 vial. Add an equal volume of trypan blue, and transfer the cell suspension to the edge of the hemocytometer chamber and it be drawn under the coverslip.
5. With a 10× objective, focus on the grid lines in the chamber, and look at the four squares at the corners of the grid. These areas are of 1 mm^2 and are the cell count areas.
6. Count the cells in this 1 mm^2 area. Do not include cells touching the lower and right limits of the square. Repeat the count for the remaining squares and sum there all. If the sample is highly concentrated, it must be diluted to obtain a final concentration of approximately 1×10^6 cells per ml.
7. Calculate the cell concentration with the following formula:

$$\text{Concentration(cell/ml)} = \frac{\text{number of cells} \times 10.000}{\text{number of squares} \times \text{dilution}}$$

8. Repeat the process up to three times with a fresh sample.

3.6 Freezing Melanoma Cells

Preserve frozen aliquots of early passage cell lines in order to prevent genetic and phenotypic instability and to avoid accidental loss of a cell line by death or contamination.

1. When cells reach confluence, gently detach the cells from tissue culture flask following the trypsinization procedure as described above.
2. Centrifuge cell suspension at 378 × *g* for 5 min at room temperature and discard supernatant. If they are at high cellular concentration, dilute cell suspension to 1×10^6 cells/ml in cold freezing media.
3. Dispense the cell suspension into pre-labeled cryotubes indicating the cell line passage number and cap them.
4. Place the cryotubes at −20 °C for 1 h.
5. Place the cryotubes at −80 °C freezer overnight.
6. Transfer the cryotubes in a cryobox to the gas phase of a liquid nitrogen freezer (−196 °C), when they reach a temperature below −50 °C (*see* **Note 13**). In the upper gas phase of liquid nitrogen freezer, they can be stored for long periods of time without appreciable cellular deterioration.

3.7 Thawing Melanoma Cells

Thawing the cells stocks, diluting the suspension, and eliminating the preservative agent must be done quickly (*see* **Note 14**).

1. In a 15 ml sterile conical tube, add 10 ml of complete DMEM medium and then take out the vial of liquid nitrogen.
2. Place the vial into a 37 °C water bath to thaw the frozen cells.
3. Once the cells are thawed, immediately clean the vial with 70% ethanol before placing it in the flow hood.
4. Transfer the thawed cell suspension into the 15 ml sterile conical tube containing 10 ml of complete medium.
5. Centrifuge at 378 × *g* for 5 min at room temperature.
6. Discard the supernatant and resuspend the pellet in fresh melanoma growth medium.
7. Transfer the cell suspension into a T-25 culture flask.
8. Incubate in a humidified atmosphere at 37 °C and 10% CO_2 overnight.
9. After 24 h check for attachment of cells to the flask, remove media and add fresh media to the flask.

3.8 Procedure to Grow Melanoma in 3D Culture by Agarose Overlay

1. Add 0.5 g of agarose to 50 ml of PBS in a 100 ml glass bottle.
2. Sterilize in autoclave to 121 °C and 15 lb/in^2 for 15 min.
3. Place 0.5 ml of the resulting solution in each of the eight-centered wells of a 24-well plate to give a base coat of 1% agarose.
4. Trypsinize the confluent melanoma primary monolayer to obtain a single-cell suspension.
5. Neutralize the trypsin with complete medium-containing FBS.
6. Calculate the cell concentration, using an electronic cell counter or a hemocytometer.
7. Place 1×10^5 cells in 500 μl of growth medium (DMEM+10% FBS) in each of the eight-centered wells of a 24-well plate, and incubate the cultures. The surrounding wells have to be filled with 1 ml of PBS in order to avoid dehydration and diminish the risk of contamination.
8. Place the plate in a CO_2 incubator. If cells are capable of spheroid formation, small aggregated clumps (about 100–300 μm in diameter) will form spontaneously in 3 to 5 days.
9. Allow the spheroids to settle, and remove single cells with the supernatant.
10. Resuspend the spheroids in fresh medium.
11. Replace the medium in the plate once or twice weekly (exchanging 0.5 ml each time), or add 300 μl of growth

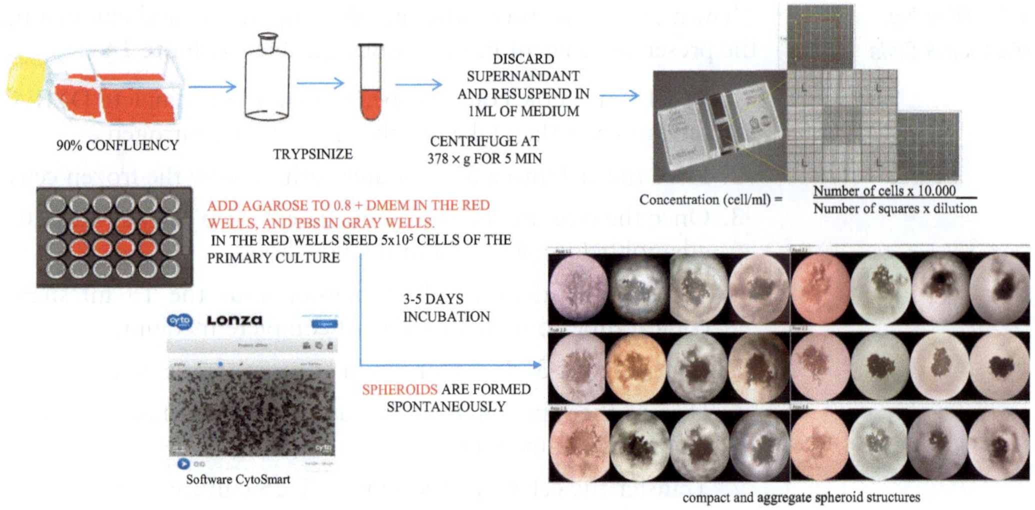

Fig. 2 Technique to obtain multicellular tumor spheroids in vitro by agarose overlay

medium (DMEM+10%FBS) in each of the eight-centered wells (without removing any medium) once or twice weekly, giving 2 ml/well after 2 to 4 weeks. (Fig. 2).

4 Notes

1. Cells were incubated with 10% instead of 5% of CO_2, to reduce the culture pH to 6.9–7.0, compared to pH 7.4–7.5 used for most cell types. This low pH concentration reduces the melanin synthesis allowing a better cell growth [16].
2. Although different media are used routinely to grow melanocytes, it is essential to consider the final tyrosine concentration in the media (10 pM tyrosine) because melanocytes convert tyrosine to melanin that can accumulate in the medium inhibiting melanoma cell growth PMID: 408156. However, we use Dulbecco's modified Eagle's medium (DMEM) which contain high levels of tyrosine (200–400 pM) and prevent the accumulation of melanin by changing the medium up to three times per week.
3. We chose to keep biopsies at room temperature and process them within the following 2 h of collection because although reports exist indicating good survival rates (at least 24 h and until 3 or 4 days) if the biopsy sample is preserved at 4 °C, we did not have satisfactory results with samples stored in refrigeration and processed the next day.
4. Biopsy decontamination is a key procedure to remove contaminating blood and to reduce surface contamination. The tissue

fragment must be large enough (200 mg or more) to be submerged in 70% ethanol without damaging the center of the tissue to isolate viable melanoma cells therefrom.

5. Specific flora of particular tissues must be taken into account in order to choose the most indicated antibiotic for each type of sample.
6. In our lab, we usually combine two or three methods for cellular disintegration depending on the nature and amount of tissue available as well as the projected use of the cells obtained. Although enzymatic digestion is labor intensive, cultures obtained by this methodology are more representative of the cells in the solid tumor in vivo.
7. The only commercial growth factor we included to obtain our cultures was insulin at a concentration of 5 μg/ml which increases the plating efficiency of several cell types. However, we obtained other non-commercial growth factors to improve melanoma growth in vitro: (1) As it has been reported that there are many potential uses of platelet-rich plasma (PRP) in tissue regeneration by inducing proliferation of a variety of human cell types in vitro [17–20], we used PRP which contain many growth factors out from the platelets such as platelet-derived growth factor (PDGF), insulin-like growth factor 1 (IGF1), and transforming growth factor (TGF) in our melanoma cell cultures. We add approximately 100,000 platelets contained in the PRP preparation. (2) Considering that melanocyte growth factors have been produced by different cell lines including melanoma and that these factors are capable to support continued proliferation of normal melanocytes [21], we reserve the first supernatant of the stablished culture, centrifuged at 1512 × *g* for 5 min, and filtered through a membrane of 0.2 μm in diameter to enrich the basal medium for melanoma used for regularly changing of culture medium.
8. Always reserve a piece of the biopsy to have a control of the original conditions of tumor microenvironment in vivo, and obtain blood samples to isolate circulating tumor cells in addition to normal PBMCs, exosomes, and molecules present in plasma. This will allow to have a broad view of tumor behavior in vivo and furthermore in vitro.
9. We chose collagenase IV due to the gentle activity of this enzyme at physiological temperature and pH that dissociates appropriately without compromising cell viability and without requirement of mechanical agitation or special equipment.
10. Although there are several protocols for decontaminate cultures which can be attempted in extreme situations, when this occurs, we always discard the culture, the medium, and reagents. At first, we applied several strategies to maintain cell

culture viability after contamination, without success. The contamination rapidly expanded leading to cell death.

11. Wash buffer to rinse away FBS which inactivate trypsin EDTA.
12. Prevent cell exposition to trypsin for longer than necessary, monitoring detachment after the first minute of trypsin exposition. Trypsin is toxic for the cells.
13. Do not submerge the cryotubes in liquid nitrogen during storage as they can take up the liquid nitrogen and explode violently on thawing.
14. Thawing frozen cells and diluting in complete DMEM medium must be done within 2 minutes after the vial removal from liquid nitrogen, because the cells will deteriorate rapidly if temperature rises above 50 °C. The initial phase of freezing and the return to normal physiological conditions are critical for cell survival.

References

1. Yamamoto Y, Ochiya T (2017) Epithelial stem cell culture: modeling human disease and applications for regenerative medicine. Inflamm Regen 37:3–10
2. Mouriaux F, Zaniolo K, Bergeron MA et al (2016) Effects of long-term serial passaging on the characteristics and properties of cell lines derived from uveal melanoma primary tumors. Invest Ophthalmol Vis Sci 57 (13):5288–5301
3. Freshney RI (2010) Culture of animal cells: a manual of basic technique and specialized applications, 6th edn. John Wiley & Sons, Inc., Hoboken, New Jersey
4. Virgone-Carlotta A, Lemasson M, Mertani HC, Diaz JJ et al (2017) In-depth phenotypic characterization of multicellular tumor spheroids: effects of 5-fluorouracil. PLoS One 12 (11):e0188100
5. Grill J, Lamfers ML, van Beusechem VW et al (2002) The organotypic multicellular spheroid is a relevant three-dimensional model to study adenovirus replication and penetration in human tumors in vitro. Mol Ther 6 (5):609–614
6. Raghavan S, Mehta P, Horst EN et al (2016) Comparative analysis of tumor spheroid generation techniques for differential in vitro drug toxicity. Oncotarget 7(13):16948–16961
7. Huanga B, Gao JQ (2018) Application of 3D cultured multicellular spheroid tumor models in tumor-targeted drug delivery system research. Bull Cancer 270:246–259
8. Vorsmann H, Groeber F, Walles H et al (2013) Development of a human three-dimensional organotypic skin-melanoma spheroid model for in vitro drug testing. Cell Death Dis 4:e719
9. Foty R (2011) A simple hanging drop cell culture protocol for generation of 3D spheroids. J Vis Exp 51:2720
10. Hirschhaeuser F, Menne H, Dittfeld C et al (2010) Multicellular tumor spheroids: an underestimated tool is catching up again. J Biotechnol 148(1):3–15
11. Coit DG, Thompson JA, Algazi A et al (2016) Melanoma, version 2 NCCN clinical practice guidelines in oncology. J Natl Compr Cancer Netw 14(4):450–473
12. Edge SB, Compton CC (2010) The American Joint Committee on Cancer: the 7th edition of the AJCC cancer staging manual and the future of TNM. Ann Surg Oncol 17(6):1471–1474
13. Halaban R, Rubin JS, Funasaka Y (1992) Met and hepatocyte growth factor/scatter factor signal transduction in normal melanocytes and melanoma cells. Oncogene 7(11):2195–2206
14. Matsumoto K, Tajima H, Nakamura T (1991) Hepatocyte growth factor is a potent stimulator of human melanocyte DNA synthesis and growth. Biochem Biophys Res Commun 176 (1):45–51

15. Yada Y, Higuchi K, Imokawa G (1991) Effects of endothelins on signal transduction and proliferation in human melanocytes. J Biol Chem 266(27):18352–18357
16. Godwin LS, Castle JT, Kohli JS (2014) Isolation, culture, and transfection of melanocytes. Curr Protoc Cell Biol 63:1–20
17. Anitua E, Andia I, Sanchez M et al (2005) Autologous preparations rich in growth factors promote proliferation and induce VEGF and HGF production by human tendon cells in culture. J Orthop Res 23(2):281–286
18. Anitua E, Sanchez M, Nurden AT et al (2007) Reciprocal actions of platelet-secreted TGF-beta1 on the production of VEGF and HGF by human tendon cells. Plast Reconstr Surg 119(3):950–959
19. Gassling VL, Acil Y, Springer IN et al (2009) Platelet-rich plasma and platelet-rich fibrin in human cell culture. Oral Surg Oral Med Oral Pathol Oral Radiol Endod 108(1):48–55
20. Li H, Usas A, Poddar M (2013) Platelet-rich plasma promotes the proliferation of human muscle derived progenitor cells and maintains their stemness. PLoS One 8(6):e64923
21. Eisinger M, Marko O, Ogata S et al (1985) Growth regulation of human melanocytes: mitogenic factors in extracts of melanoma, astrocytoma, and fibroblast cell lines. Science 229(4717):984–986

Chapter 9

Assessment of Antitumor T-Cell Responses by Flow Cytometry After Coculture of Tumor Cells with Autologous Tumor-Infiltrating Lymphocytes

Jeroen Melief, Stina Wickström, Rolf Kiessling, and Yago Pico de Coaña

Abstract

As a consequence of the ever-increasing use of immunotherapy for the treatment of cancer, interest in the direct interaction between T cells and tumors has surged tremendously. In vitro coculture of tumor cells with autologous tumor-infiltrating lymphocytes (TIL) is a highly physiological and clinically relevant model to study functional T-cell responses that result from the array of activatory and inhibitory signals that naturally occur on the patient's own tumor cells. This chapter describes a detailed protocol to set up a tumor-TIL coculture and assess ensuing functional T-cell responses, in order to establish the strength of tumor recognition by T cells and identify key determinants that govern this.

Key words T cells, Tumor-infiltrating lymphocytes (TIL), Tumor cells, Immunotherapy, Tumor immunology

1 Introduction

The recent years have seen a large increase in immunotherapeutic approaches for cancer, with notable clinical success being achieved by checkpoint blockade and cellular therapies [1]. By far the large majority of cancer immunotherapies in use or in clinical development aim to promote T cell-mediated tumor eradication. Therefore, the success of these approaches critically depends on the extent to which T cells are able to identify their appropriate target cells through antigen recognition in the context of a variety of inhibitory and activatory signals [2, 3].

Importantly, the total sum of activatory and inhibitory signals detected on a target cell determines whether T-cell activation and cytotoxicity will actually occur [4]. In vitro coculture of tumor cells with autologous tumor-infiltrating lymphocytes (TIL) is widely seen as the most suitable tool to study this in a physiologically and clinically relevant way, as it measures functional T-cell responses

Yago Pico de Coaña (ed.), *Immune Checkpoint Blockade: Methods and Protocols*, Methods in Molecular Biology, vol. 1913, https://doi.org/10.1007/978-1-4939-8979-9_9, © Springer Science+Business Media, LLC, part of Springer Nature 2019

that result from recognition of all the activatory and inhibitory signals that naturally occur on the patient's own tumor cells. As such, the model gives insight into the intrinsic abilities of T cells to detect autologous cancer cells in specific patients or even in specific areas of a tumor.

Other, more experimental questions can be addressed by manipulating cells prior to their use in a coculture. For example, tumor cells can be pretreated with immunostimulatory agents or chemotherapeutic compounds to assess their effect on tumor immunogenicity. Similarly, TIL may be sorted, for example according to phenotypic markers or antigen specificity, to study antitumor responses of T-cell subpopulations in more detail. During the actual coculture, molecular interactions between effector and target cells may be blocked by antibodies (e.g., for PD-1) to study their individual role in promoting or suppressing antitumor T-cell responses. In all cases, any tumor-TIL coculture should always include wells without any target cells. The T cells in these wells should be cultured alone or in the presence of activation beads coated with anti-CD3/CD28 antibodies, which, respectively, serve as a negative and positive control to get insight into baseline and maximal levels of T-cell activation in the particular batch or vial of cells used in the assay.

In this chapter we describe a detailed protocol with the steps required to set up a tumor-TIL coculture and assess ensuing functional T-cell responses. Several readout techniques may be used to assess T-cell responses in the tumor-TIL coculture, including ELISA and flow cytometry. To determine T-cell activation, cytokine levels (e.g. of interleukin-2 or interferon-gamma) in the supernatants of these cocultures may be measured by ELISA, which serves as a less laborious and costly readout that may be more suitable for experiments with many conditions, including larger-scale screenings. The main readout on which we focus in this chapter describes staining the cocultured cells with fluorescently labeled antibodies and analyzing them by flow cytometry. In this setting, flow cytometry will give most detailed information as it provides a phenotypic characterization of the cells involved in the response in combination with two indicators of functional T-cell activation, such as CD107a for degranulation [5], and the production of IFN-γ, which is the hallmark cytokine produced by T cells in an antitumor response [6].

2 Materials

2.1 Cells

1. Purified T cells (*see* **Note 1**).
2. Target tumor cell line (*see* **Note 2**).

2.2 General

1. General cell culture equipment and plastics such as pipettes, tips, tubes, etc.
2. LAF-bench.
3. Cell culture incubator set at 37 °C, 5% CO_2.
4. Centrifuge with swing-out rotor.
5. Microscope.
6. Inverted microscope.
7. Cell counter or counting chamber for manual counting.
8. Phosphate buffered saline (PBS) pH 7.4: 137 mM NaCl, 2.7 mM KCl, 10 mM $Na_2HPO_4 \times 2H_2O$, 2 mM KH_2PO_4.

2.3 T Cell: Tumor Cell Line Coculture

1. 96-well plates (*see* **Notes 3** and **4**).
2. Coculture medium: RPMI medium, 2% human AB serum.
3. LEAF™ Purified antihuman HLA-A, HLA-B, HLA-C [W6/32] (BioLegend) (*see* **Note 5**).
4. Dynabeads Human T-Activator CD3/CD28 (Life Technologies).

2.4 Intracellular Staining and Flow Cytometry

1. 96-well V-bottom plates.
2. Aqua Dead Cell Marker (AquaDCM): LIVE/DEAD™ Fixable Aqua Dead Cell Stain Kit, for 405 nm excitation (Thermo Fisher Scientific) (*see* **Note 6**).
3. IVIg 100 mg ml (Privigen) (*see* **Note** 7).
4. Antibodies for flow cytometry: Anti human CD8 APC-Cy7, CD3 PE-Cy7, IFN-γ PE, CD107a FITC.
5. Fixation/Permeabilization Solution Kit (BD Biosciences).
6. BD GolgiPlug™ Protein Transport Inhibitor (containing brefeldin A) (BD Biosciences).
7. BD GolgiStop™ Protein Transport Inhibitor (containing monensin) (BD Biosciences).
8. Flow cytometer with at least seven channels (FSC, SSC + 5) (*see* **Note 8**).
9. Computer with appropriate software for flow cytometry analysis (*see* **Note 9**).

3 Methods

3.1 T Cell-Tumor Cell Line Coculture

1. Thaw the vials of T cells to be tested in a 37 °C water bath.
2. Transfer the contents of each vial to a 50 ml falcon tube with 10 ml coculture medium.
3. Count T cells, and centrifuge 5 min at 350 × *g* (*see* **Note 10**).

4. Resuspend in coculture medium at a final concentration of 2×10^6 cells/ml.
5. Harvest tumor cells and transfer into a 50 ml falcon tube (*see* **Note 11**).
6. Centrifuge 5 min at $350 \times g$.
7. Resuspend in 5 ml coculture medium. Count cells (*see* **Note 10**).
8. Transfer the needed number of tumor cells to an additional falcon tube, and add PBS to a final concentration of 2×10^6 cells/ml.
9. Plate 25 μl tumor cells per well (50,000 cells) in a 96-well round-bottom plate (*see* **Note 12**).
10. Dilute antihuman HLA-A, HLA-B, and HLA-C antibody to 40 μg/ml. Add 25 μl to the appropriate well (*see* **Note 13**).
11. Incubate 30 min at 37 °C.
12. Add 4 μl CD107a-FITC antibody to each well (*see* **Notes 14** and **15**).
13. Add 50 μl (100,000 cells) TIL per well (*see* **Note 12**).
14. Dilute CD3/CD28 Dynabeads: 2 μl + 48 μl coculture medium.
15. Add 25 μl CD3/CD28 mix to the appropriate well.
16. Adjust the volume of all wells to 104 μl with coculture medium (*see* **Note 16**).
17. Incubate plate 2 h at 37 °C.
18. Prepare protein transport inhibitor solution: 145 μl coculture medium, 3 μl GolgiPlug and 2 μl GolgiStop. Add 5 μl/well.
19. Incubate plate 4 h at 37 °C.
20. Collect supernatant and freeze at −20 °C (*see* **Note 17**).
21. Transfer cells to a 96-well V-bottom plate.
22. Centrifuge 3 min at $700 \times g$, 4 °C and proceed to intracellular cytokine staining.

3.2 Intracellular Cytokine Staining

1. Add 200 μl PBS, and centrifuge 3 min at $700 \times g$, 4 °C. Repeat wash step (*see* **Notes 18** and **19**).
2. Prepare DCM: 1 μl stock +1000 μl PBS. Add 200 μl/sample. Panels 1, 2, 3, and 5 are stained with AquaDCM. Incubate 10–15 min at 4 °C protected from light (*see* **Note 20**).
3. Make a mix of 12 μl CD8 APC-Cy7 (1.5 μl/sample),4 μl CD3 PE-Cy7 (0.5 μl/sample) and 144 μl FACS buffer (*see* **Note 21**). Add 20 μl per well.
4. Incubate at 4 °C protected from light for 20 min.

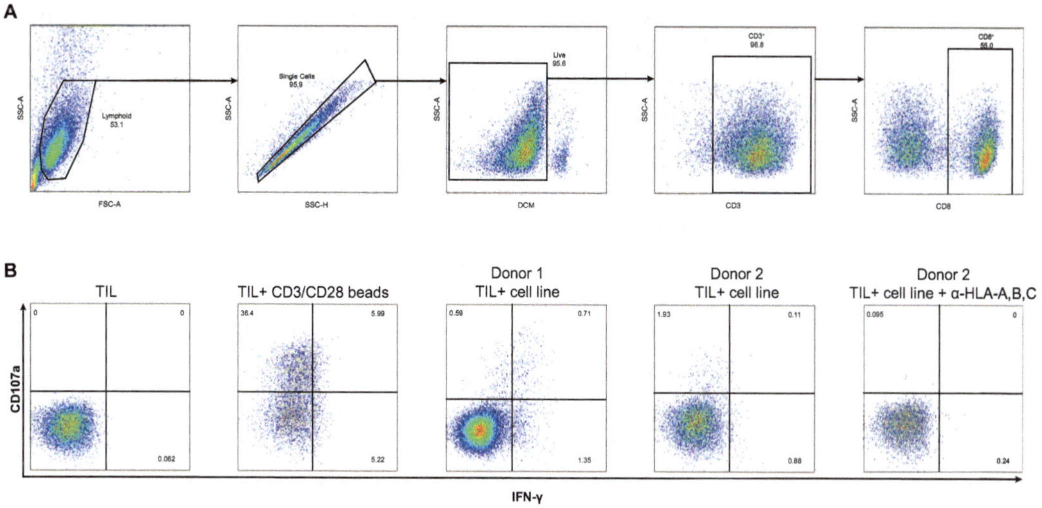

Fig. 1 Gating strategy and reactivity analysis. (**a**) Gating strategy for CD3^{+} CD8^{+} T cell determination. (**b**) Sample results for controls and two assays corresponding to TIL-cell line pairs from different donors

5. After extracellular staining is complete, add 200 μl FACS buffer to each well and centrifuge 3 min at 700 × *g*, 4 °C. Repeat wash step.
6. Add 100 μl fixation/permeabilization solution and incubate 15–20 min at 4 °C.
7. After the permeabilization incubation time has ended, wash the plate twice with 200 μl BD Perm/Wash buffer (centrifuge at 700 × *g*, 3 min, 4 °C).
8. Make a mix of 32 μl IFN-γ PE and 128 μl FACS PermWash. Add 20 μl per well (*see* **Note 21**) and incubate for 40 min at 4 °C protected from light.
9. Wash once with 200 μl diluted PermWash and once with FACS buffer.
10. Resuspend in 200 μl FACS buffer and acquire on flow cytometer.
11. Analyze data. Initially debris, dead cells, and doublets will be excluded. In a second step, CD3^{+} CD8^{+} T cells are selected (Fig. 1a). Tumor recognition is determined comparing the frequencies of IFN-γ^{+}, CD107a^{+}, and double positive cells with the negative and positive controls (*see* **Note 22**).

4 Notes

1. In addition to TIL, the T cells to be used in this assay can also be T cells purified from circulating blood or other tissues. Furthermore, prior to their use in coculture with tumor cells, purified T cells may be sorted additionally into subpopulations,

for example, according to lineage and/or differentiation markers or antigen-specificity. Another possibility is to label T cells with CFSE, which can be detected by flow cytometry to determine cell proliferation.

2. Tumor cells can be pretreated with immunostimulatory agents, such as interferon-gamma (IFN-γ), or chemotherapeutic or targeted compounds, to assess their effect on tumor immunogenicity. Wash tumor cells properly before start of the coculture to ensure complete removal of the agent used for pretreatment.
3. Most suitable are U-bottom plates, but flat-bottom plates will also work.
4. A standard assay should always include the following wells, which should be run in duplicate:
   (a) Unstimulated T cells as a negative control.
   (b) T cells stimulated with CD3/CD28 Dynabeads as a positive control.
   (c) T cells + cell line + antihuman HLA-A, HLA-B, HLA-C, to block T-cell recognition as a negative control.
   (d) T cells + cell line.
5. This antibody should always be used to assess whether target cell recognition is antigen-mediated. Other blocking antibodies may be used to study additional molecular interactions between effector and target cells for their role in antitumor T-cell responses. Make sure antibodies are suitable for applications with living cells, such as the low-endotoxin azide-free (LEAF) antibody used here.
6. We dissolve the original reagent in 50 μl of the provided DMSO and then make 1 μl aliquots in brown Eppendorf tubes, which can be used directly for compensation or frozen and diluted 1:1000 in PBS to stain samples when needed.
7. We use IVIg as an Fc receptor blocking reagent. Other blocking reagents work equally well.
8. We use a BD LSRII with the configuration shown in Table 1. The staining panel was created for this flow cytometer.
9. We currently use FlowJo v10 (FlowJo, LLC, USA).
10. In case several cell suspensions are prepared that were, for example, subjected to sorting or pretreatment protocols, apply a reliable counting method to ensure equal amounts of cells are used in the coculture.
11. If the cell line is to be kept in culture, reseed leftover cells in an appropriate flask. Otherwise freeze or discard as needed.
12. The number of cells used may be varied based on the sensitivity of the target cell to recognition by the T cells used for coculture. The most commonly used effector:target (E:T) ratio is 2:1.

Table 1
BD Biosciences LSRII flow cytometer configuration

Laser name	Wavelength	Detector array	Detector	Channel	Mirror	Filter	Parameter
Blue	488	Octagon	A	5	735 LP	780/60 BP	PE-Cy7
			B	4	680 LP	712/21 BP	PerCP-Cy5-5
			C	3	635 LP	670/14 BP	PerCP
			D	2	595 LP	610/20 BP	PE-CF594
			E	13	555 LP	575/26 BP	PE
			F	12	505 LP	530/30 BP	FITC
			G	1		488/10 BP	SSC
Violet	407	Trigon	A	7	555 LP	585/42 BP	Pacific Orange
			B	6	505 LP	525/50 BP	Aqua DCM
			C	14		450/50 BP	Pacific Blue
325 UV	325	Trigon	B	8	505 LP	450/50 BP	DAPI
Red	633	Trigon	A	11	735 LP	780/60 BP	APC-Cy7
			C	15		660/20 BP	APC
							Alexa Fluor 647

13. At this point, also dilute any other blocking antibodies of potential interest to achieve the desired end concentration in the well.
14. The amount of this antibody, as well as the other antibodies used in this protocol, should be properly titrated before use.
15. Also include wells with only T cells that are not stained for CD107a, to determine the background signal for this marker.
16. It is easier to make the appropriate calculations beforehand, taking into account which well contains each of the necessary elements for the experiment: cancer cells, T cells, CD3/CD28 Dynabeads, and blocking antibodies.
17. Supernatant may be used at a later point to detect levels of IFN-γ as a measure of T-cell activation by ELISA. If ELISA is used as the sole readout, it is recommended to incubate the coculture for 24 h to allow IFN-γ secreted by T cells to accumulate in the supernatant to levels that can be detected more readily. IFN-γ (or other relevant cytokine) concentration in these supernatants can be measured using readily available commercial cytokine quantitation ELISA kits.
18. Discard supernatant in a single swift motion. Repeatedly tipping the plate will result in pellets becoming dislodged.

19. It is essential to wash cells in PBS without any type of human or bovine protein, as this will bind to the DCM and reduce its ability to stain nonviable cells.
20. During staining, it is essential to protect fluorescent reagents and conjugated antibodies from light. We recommend turning off the lights in the flow hood. Additionally, tandem-conjugated antibodies are sensitive to temperature. The ideal setting for undisturbed incubations in the dark and at 4 °C is a lidded styrofoam box half full with ice.
21. This mix is calculated to stain eight samples. It can be stored at 4 °C for up to 2 weeks.
22. In this chapter we have used IFN-γ release and CD107a^{+} as the standard functional markers for CD8 T-cell activation. Depending on the different hypothesis to be tested, additional cytokines (such as TNF-α or IL-2) and activation markers can also be analyzed.

References

1. Yang Y (2015) Cancer immunotherapy: harnessing the immune system to battle cancer. J Clin Invest 125(9):3335–3337. https://doi.org/10.1172/JCI83871
2. Pardoll DM (2012) The blockade of immune checkpoints in cancer immunotherapy. Nat Rev Cancer 12(4):252–264. https://doi.org/10.1038/nrc3239
3. Prajapati K, Perez C, Rojas LBP, Burke B, Guevara-Patino JA (2018) Functions of NKG2D in CD8(+) T cells: an opportunity for immunotherapy. Cell Mol Immunol. https://doi.org/10.1038/cmi.2017.161
4. Blankenstein T, Coulie PG, Gilboa E, Jaffee EM (2012) The determinants of tumour immunogenicity. Nat Rev Cancer 12(4):307–313. https://doi.org/10.1038/nrc3246
5. Betts MR, Brenchley JM, Price DA, De Rosa SC, Douek DC, Roederer M et al (2003) Sensitive and viable identification of antigen-specific CD8 + T cells by a flow cytometric assay for degranulation. J Immunol Methods 281(1–2):65–78
6. Schroder K, Hertzog PJ, Ravasi T, Hume DA (2004) Interferon-gamma: an overview of signals, mechanisms and functions. J Leukoc Biol 75(2):163–189. https://doi.org/10.1189/jlb.0603252

Chapter 10

Expansion and Determination of Antigen-Reactive T Cells by Flow Cytometry

Alexander Martens, Graham Pawelec, and Christopher Shipp

Abstract

The detection of antigen-reactive T cells has shown great utility for patient clinical monitoring. However, many of the methods commonly used to detect these cells face major limitations, like the predetermination of the given HLA type. The herein described protocol provides a means of overcoming many of the obstacles associated with the use of multimers and other common approaches in this field. In order to be able to detect rare cells which are below the detection limit of direct ex vivo measurement, in the present protocol, antigen-reactive T cells are first expanded in vitro using libraries of overlapping peptides which span the entire protein of interest and consist of 15 amino acid-long peptides that share a 12-amino-acid overlap. This theoretically allows the detection of T cells to any epitope within a protein of interest and consequently does not require the patient's HLA type to be characterized. Furthermore, this method simultaneously detects CD4+ and CD8+ T cells that produce cytokines upon encounter with antigen and thereby provides a functional insight into the behavior of the responding T cells. In our case, we have investigated the pro- or anti-inflammatory cytokines IL-2, IL-5, IL-10, IL-17, TNF-α, and IFN-γ.

Key words Antigen-reactive T cells, Overlapping peptides, Tumor-associated antigen, Intracellular cytokine staining, Clinical monitoring, Flow cytometry

1 Introduction

The emergence of modern flow cytometers has resulted in the widespread use of multi-parametric flow cytometry in clinical research. Due to its ability to simultaneously provide information from a large number of different cell types or proteins, this technology is commonly used for the clinical monitoring of patients with cancer. This approach has uncovered clinically relevant biomarkers from the peripheral blood of patients with melanoma [1], lung [2], prostate [3], renal [4], and many other types of cancer [5]. Many of these studies employ immunophenotyping of immune cell populations in general; however, this technology is also able to detect specific populations of antigen-reactive T cells. Given that tumor control is largely mediated by T cells recognizing tumor

Yago Pico de Coaña (ed.), *Immune Checkpoint Blockade: Methods and Protocols*, Methods in Molecular Biology, vol. 1913, https://doi.org/10.1007/978-1-4939-8979-9_10, © Springer Science+Business Media, LLC, part of Springer Nature 2019

antigens, assessing these cells is also useful in identifying clinically relevant immune parameters in cancer patients [4, 6–8].

Because many of the common approaches used to detect antigen-reactive T cells are associated with a number of restrictions, alternative methods overcoming these limitations may be more widely implementable and more informative than current approaches. Multimer technology, such as tetramers, has traditionally been popular for the detection of antigen-reactive T cells. Despite its popularity, this method has major drawbacks; it requires the antigenic epitope to be known and consequently for each patient's MHC type to be characterized. This reduces the practicality and increases the cost of this method, but it additionally means that only T cells specific for a particular epitope can be detected at a time. A further obstacle to the detection of antigen-reactive T cells using ex vivo approaches such as multimers is the low frequency of antigen-specific T cells in the peripheral blood, which is estimated to fall in the range of 0.0001–0.1% of T cells [9]. This may be overcome by enriching the cell type of interest, but in turn this necessitates that larger quantities of patient material must be available. The protocol reported here is not bound by these limiting factors due to the employment of in vitro stimulation prior to the detection of antigen-reactive T cells. Stimulation is performed with pools of peptides covering the entire protein sequence of the selected target molecule, consequently eliminating the requirement for epitope prediction and patient HLA typing. In the examples referred to in this chapter, peptide pools were used that consist of a mix of 15 amino acid (AA)-long peptides with a 12 AA overlap. Furthermore, this approach theoretically allows the detection of T cells recognizing the entire potential antigenic repertoire, i.e., every possible epitope that could be generated from the target molecule. Prior in vitro stimulation allows an assessment of the functional state of reactive T cells by measuring their cytokine production pattern upon encounter with antigen, assesses the patient's antigen presentation capacity, and also may further reduce the requirement for patient material.

This approach has revealed specific populations of antigen-reactive T cells that represent biomarkers correlating with patient survival in melanoma and breast cancer [7, 10, 11]. This method uses multi-parameter flow cytometry to determine (1) whether a given patient possesses CD4+ or CD8+ T cells reactive to a particular antigen and (2) the cytokine production profile of such reactive T cells. Because this approach provides a functional understanding of both CD4+ and CD8+ T cells producing pro- or anti-inflammatory cytokines, it may be more accurate in the identification of clinically important immune responses.

2 Materials

1. Serum-free cell culture medium: X-VIVO 15.
2. RPMI: RPMI medium 1640 (1×) (containing GlutaMax).
3. PBS: Dulbecco's phosphate-buffered saline.
4. Pepmix: 1 μg/mL of each peptide per test (*see* **Note 1**).
5. IL-2: 40 U/mL in X-VIVO 15. Dilute 2 μL of the stock solution (1 × 10^6 U/mL) in 1998 μL X-VIVO 15. Take 80 μL of the diluted stock, and dilute this into another 920 μL medium to reach a concentration of 80 U/mL. The final concentration of IL-2 in the cell culture well is reached by adding the diluted IL-2 to an equal volume of medium.
6. IL-4: 5 ng/mL diluted in X-VIVO 15.
7. IL-7: 5 ng/mL diluted in X-VIVO 15.
8. GolgiPlug: 1 × GolgiPlug in X-VIVO 15. In the current protocol, GolgiPlug was diluted 1:1000 prior to use (i.e., 1 μL in 1 mL). Prepare a 3× GolgiPlug solution in X-VIVO 15 immediately prior to usage, e.g., 30 μL GolgiPlug in a total of 10 mL X-VIVO 15, depending on the number of samples to be tested.
9. Flow cytometry staining buffer (PFEA): 2% FCS, 2 mM EDTA, and 0.01% NaN_3 (diluted in 1 × PBS). Add 10 mL FCS, 2 mL 500 mM EDTA, and 50 mg NaN_3 to 500 mL 1 × PBS. Store at 4 °C.
10. Fc blocking reagent: 10% Gamunex in 900 μL PFEA.
11. Live dead staining: 1 μg/mL ethidium monoazide (EMA).
12. Cytofix/Cytoperm: As directed by the manufacturer.
13. Perm/Wash: 1× Perm/Wash in ddH_2O.

3 Methods

All cell culture steps to expand antigen-reactive T cells should be carried out at RT (room temperature) under a sterile bench. Ensure all reagents that come in contact with cells are sterile and intended for use in cell culture.

3.1 Thawing of PBMCs

1. Thaw ampoules of cryopreserved PBMCs in a preheated 37 °C water bath (*see* **Note 2**).
2. Label centrifuge tubes, and add 4 °C RPMI medium before or while PBMCs are thawing. The volume of RPMI to be added should be equal to the volume in the cryopreserved PBMC ampoule (*see* **Note 3**).

3. Invert the ampoule several times, and transfer the entire volume into the prepared centrifuged tubes containing RPMI.
4. Shake carefully to mix before incubating for 5 min at RT.
5. Following this incubation step, add the same volume of RPMI once more, and centrifuge for 10 min at 200 × *g*.
6. Discard the supernatant by carefully inverting the tube before resuspending the cells in 1 mL of RT cell culture medium (X-VIVO 15).
7. Count the PBMCs, and adjust the volume to reach a concentration of 8 × 10^6 PBMCs/mL.
8. Supplement the culture medium with IL-4 (5 ng/mL) and IL-7 (5 ng/mL). It is recommended to use at least 1 × 10^6 PBMCs per antigen of interest.

3.2 Expansion of Antigen-Reactive T Cells

1. Day 0: A minimum of 2 × 10^6 PBMCs are required per donor. 1 × 10^6 PBMCs are seeded and expanded with peptides derived from the antigen(s) of interest, e.g., tumor-associated antigens. A further 1 × 10^6 PBMCs are required as an experimental control; these cells are seeded in separate wells from those to be stimulated with the antigen of interest. Control antigens, for example, from influenza viruses for which most individuals are expected to have prior exposure, are used as a positive biological control to test whether the cells are functional. If the investigation will employ testing of more than one antigen of interest, the number of cells required, medium volume and tissue culture plate should be adjusted accordingly (*see* Table 1 and **Notes 4** and **5**).
2. Transfer 1 × 10^6 PBMCs per antigen into the appropriate tissue culture-treated plates (flat bottom). Allow cells to rest overnight in an incubator (37 °C, 5% CO_2, 95% humidity in air).
3. Day 1: Add an equal volume of cell culture media containing IL-4 (5 ng/mL) and IL-7 (5 ng/mL) to each well.
4. The PBMCs are then stimulated by adding 1 μg/mL (10 μL/mL) of peptide (per antigen) to the wells. As previously mentioned, stimulation by peptides derived from different antigens of interest can be performed in the same well, but stimulation with control peptides should be carried out in a separate well.
5. Day 3: Remove half of the well volume, and re-add the same volume of fresh culture medium supplemented with IL-2 at a final concentration of 40 U/mL (*see* **Note 6**).
6. Day 4–11: On day 3, add freshly prepared cell culture media containing IL-2 to every well.

Table 1
Required number of cells, medium volume, and tissue culture plate type depending on the number of antigens to be tested

Number of antigens of interest	Total volume on day 0	Number of PBMCs	Size of tissue culture plate
1[a]	125 μL	1×10^6	96 well plate
2	250 μL	2×10^6	48 well plate
3	375 μL	3×10^6	24 well plate
4	500 μL	4×10^6	24 well plate

[a]Control peptides are cultured in the same setup

7. Subsequent to day 3, replace depleted cell culture medium in every well of the plate when medium becomes depleted (i.e., when the culture media changes color from red to orange) by removing half of the volume and re-adding the same volume together with freshly prepared IL-2.
8. Repeat this procedure as necessary (*see* **Notes** 7 and **8**).

3.3 Restimulation of Expanded Antigen-Reactive T Cells

1. Day 12: Carefully resuspend cells, and transfer the contents of each well into a separate 15 mL centrifuge tube.
2. Add 5 mL of RPMI and centrifuge for 10 min at 200 × *g* at RT.
3. Discard the supernatant (this step is performed to remove any IL-2, IL-4, or IL-7 that may remain).
4. Count the cells (a minimum of 500,000 cells per antigen is recommended), and resuspend them in the required volume of fresh culture medium (*see* **Note 9**).
5. Equally distribute the contents into the necessary number of wells in a 96-well round-bottom tissue culture plate (*see* Tables 2 and 3 and Fig. 1—e.g., cells from three antigens of interest that were previously cultured in a single well should now be split into three separate wells for each antigen, plus an additional well as an unstimulated control) (*see* **Note 10**).
6. Add 100 μL of 3 × concentrated GolgiPlug and 1 μg/mL of the respective pepmix to each well to be restimulated, (i.e., 3 μL of the previously diluted pepmix) so that the total volume of each well is 300 μL (*see* **Note 11**). Extra caution should be taken so that each well only contains the indicated peptide and that the non-restimulated controls do not contain any peptide.
7. Incubate overnight for 12 h at 37 °C, 5% CO_2, and 20% O_2 (*see* **Note 12**).

Table 2
Required medium volume and number of wells for control antigen restimulation

Number of control antigens	Minimal total volume of fresh X-VIVO 15	Total number and volume of wells[a]
1	400 μL	2 × 200 μL

[a]The final volume of each well will be 300 μL after the addition of peptide and GolgiPlug

Table 3
Required medium volume and number of wells for restimulation with antigens of interest

Number of antigens of interest	Minimal total volume of fresh X-VIVO 15	Total number of wells
1	400 μL	2 × 200 μL
2	600 μL	3 × 200 μL
3	800 μL	4 × 200 μL
4	1000 μL	5 × 200 μL

The final volume of each well will be 300 μL after the addition of peptide and GolgiPlug

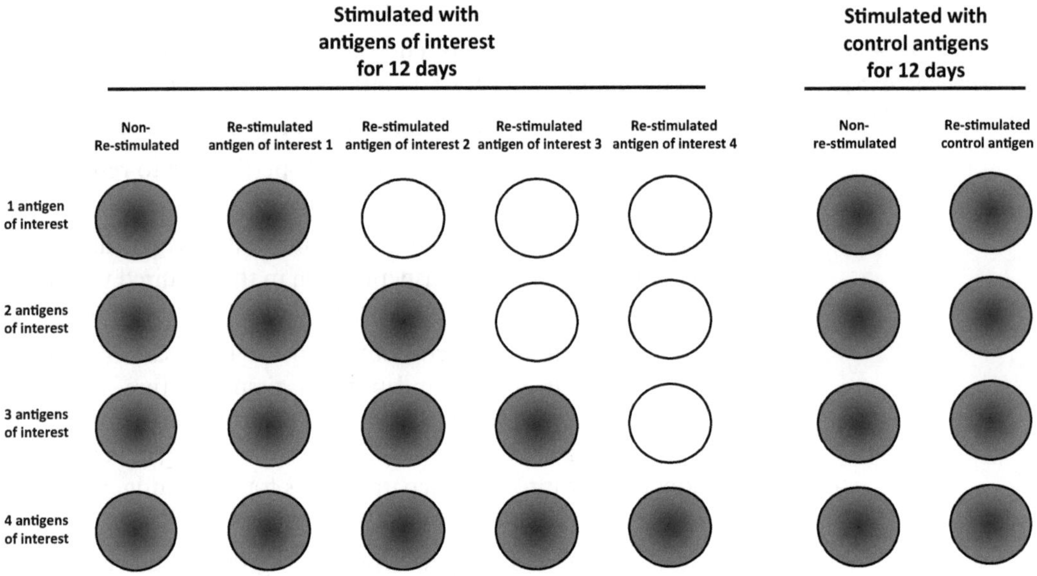

Fig. 1 Example pipetting scheme for peptide restimulation. The example scheme depicts the required number of wells for restimulation whether 1, 2, 3, or 4 antigens of interest (left) and respective control antigens (right) are assessed. Darkened circles indicate the presence of cells, and unfilled circles indicate empty wells

3.4 Intracellular Antibody Staining

1. Following 12 h of peptide stimulation, resuspend cells, and transfer PBMCs from the respective wells into flow cytometry sample tubes.

Table 4
Example flow cytometry antibody panel to assess antigen-reactive T cells

Antibody	Fluorochrome	Clone
CD3	PO	UCHT
CD4	PB	RPA-T4
CD8	APC-H7	SK1
IL-2	A700	MQ1-17H12
IL-5	PE	JES1-39D10
IL-10	APC	JES3-9D7
IL-17	PerCP-Cy5.5	eBio64DEC17
TNF-α	FITC	MAb11
IFN-γ	PE-Cy7	B27

2. All incubation steps for flow cytometry should be performed on ice. Resuspend the transferred cells in 1 mL PFEA staining buffer to dilute the remaining cell culture media.
3. Centrifuge for 5 min at 300 × *g* and 4 °C and discard the supernatant.
4. Block Fc receptors to avoid nonspecific antibody binding with 50 μL of the diluted Fc blocking reagent.
5. Simultaneously label nonviable cells with 1 μL of the live/dead cell marker.
6. Incubate for 20 min under a bright fluorescent light source.
7. After the incubation period, add 1 mL of PFEA and centrifuge for 5 min at 300 × *g* and discard supernatant.
8. Resuspend cells in 100 μL of Cytofix/Cytoperm solution.
9. Incubate for 20 min on ice in the dark.
10. Resuspend cells in 1 mL Perm/Wash, and centrifuge for 5 min at 300 × *g* and discard supernatant.
11. Repeat. Resuspend cells in 1 mL Perm/Wash and incubate for 15 min in the dark.
12. Centrifuge for 5 min at 300 × *g* and discard supernatant.
13. Prepare a mastermix (*see* Table 4) with all antibodies, and add 50 μL to each sample (*see* **Notes 13** and **14**).
14. Incubate for 30 min in the dark.
15. After the incubation period, resuspend cells in 1 mL Perm/Wash, and centrifuge for 5 min at 300 × *g* and discard supernatant.

16. Repeat this washing step before resuspending cells in 100 μL of PFEA.
17. Measure samples with a flow cytometer within 4 h of completing the staining procedure. In the current protocol, a 14-color BD LSR II flow cytometer was employed.

3.5 Determination of Antigen-Reactive T Cells

The following rules have been established to determine whether T cells are reactive to a certain antigen or not:

1. T cells are considered reactive to an antigen if the CD4+ or CD8+ T cells from the donor produce at least one of the following six cytokines (IL-2, IL-5, IL-10, IL-17, TNF-α, IFN-γ) upon restimulation with the antigen of interest.
2. The frequency of cytokine-positive cells has to be at least twofold over the non-restimulated control (*see* **Note 15**).
3. A distinct population of cytokine-producing cells has to be present.
4. The T cells stimulated with control peptides have to be positive according to rules 1–3.

Figure 2 shows examples of a patient sample positive for antigen-reactive T cells. The herein described protocol could theoretically be modified to investigate many different types of proteins produced by T cells upon antigen encounter.

4 Notes

1. Consult the peptide manufacturer for the required handling and storage procedure. The pepmixes used in this protocol were first dissolved in 40 μL pure DMSO and then further diluted in 210 μL PBS. This was then aliquoted into 25 vials (each 10 μL) and stored at −20 °C. Avoid multiple freezing and thawing cycles.
2. We suggest Wednesday as the most convenient day to thaw and seed PBMC samples. If two seeding days per week are required, we suggest Wednesday and Friday as the most convenient days to minimize work over the weekends.
3. To increase the recovery rate and to reduce the exposure time to the DMSO-containing medium used to cryopreserve the cells, remove the ampoule of PBMCs from the water bath when a small clump of ice is still present.
4. PBMCs can be pooled and stimulated with multiple antigens of interest in the same well, resulting in reduced tissue culture work.

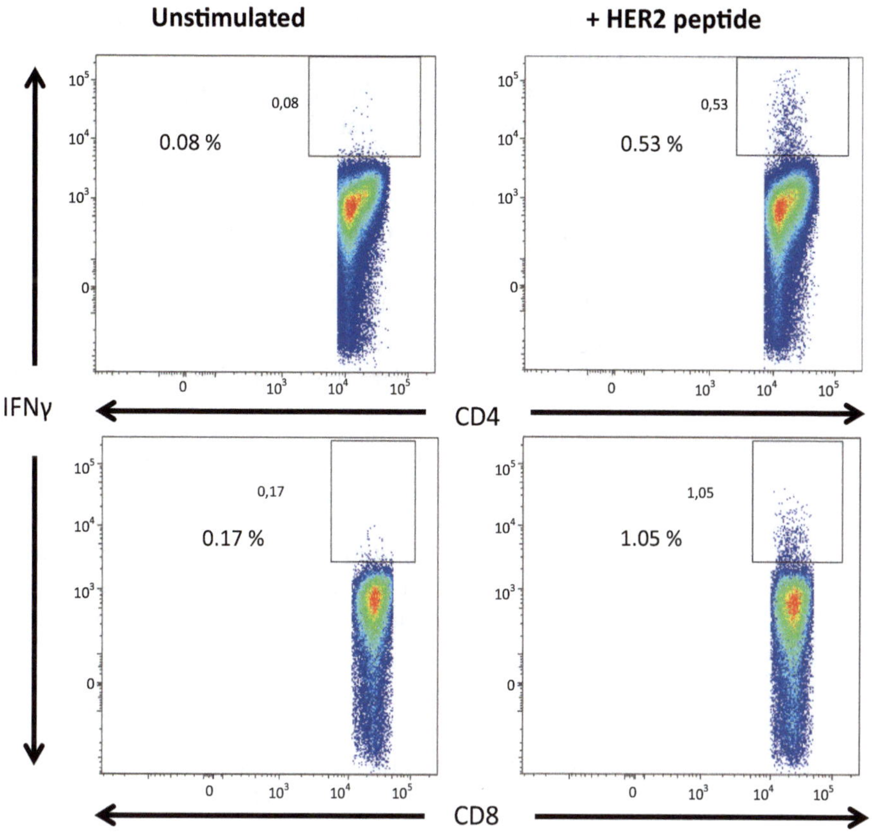

Fig. 2 Example of a positive T cell response upon peptide restimulation. The figure shows a patient who possesses CD4+ (upper panel) and CD8+ (lower panel) T cells positive for IFN-gamma when stimulated with the HER2 antigen. Note the distinct population of cytokine-producing cells in response to the peptide that is more than twice the frequency of cytokine-producing cells in the non-restimulated control without peptide. Image obtained from [12]

5. Based on our experience, the simultaneous testing of up to six different patient samples for four antigens of interest and one control antigen is feasible for a single person. This includes the required tissue culture work, antibody staining and flow cytometric measurements.
6. Diluted IL-2 solution should always be prepared freshly from a stock solution before use. Undiluted stock may be stored at 4 °C for 1 month.
7. The total volume of the wells may vary due to evaporation, particularly for wells located on the outer edge of cell culture plates. This effect can be reduced by adding medium to any empty wells present in the culture plate.
8. The exchange of tissue culture medium should be performed for every well in the plate, regardless of the appearance of the

medium, to ensure consistency in the treatment of separate wells.

9. Carefully resuspend the volume with a pipette to ensure a homogeneous and equal distribution in all wells of the tissue culture plate.
10. If it is intended to restimulate and later measure reactivity to multiple antigens but the required cell number per antigen of interest is not met, reduce the number of antigens to be restimulated based on your personal priority.
11. The 96 well plates can be centrifuged for several seconds at $200 \times g$ to accumulate cells at the bottom of the wells.
12. If it is not possible to start with the antibody staining after the 12 h of incubation have passed, it is possible to store the plate for additional time at 4 °C. We have tested up to but not beyond 2 h storage poststimulation. Alternatively, the stimulation period may be extended – we have tested up to a maximum of 14 h. Note that we recommend all samples from a single study to be consistent in terms of the peptide stimulation period used.
13. Certain cell surface marker antibodies may be recommended by the manufacturer to be incubated with cells that are not permeabilized. In this case, these antibodies may need to be incubated prior to permeabilization. Be sure to read the technical data sheet of each antibody.
14. Antibody concentrations should be selected after performing a titration. Once optimal concentrations are determined, the antibody mastermix should be made up by diluting the required volume of each antibody in Perm/Wash (or in PFEA if the antibodies are to be applied prior to permeabilization). Fluorescence minus one (FMO) controls are additionally recommended to test the compatibility of separate antibodies used in the same panel.
15. Measure non-restimulated samples before restimulated samples to avoid the potential of sample cross-contamination, as the population of cytokine-producing cells is usually very small (below 1% of the total population).

References

1. Martens A, Wistuba-Hamprecht K, Geukes Foppen M, Yuan J, Postow MA, Wong P, Romano E, Khammari A, Dreno B, Capone M, Ascierto PA, Di Giacomo AM, Maio M, Schilling B, Sucker A, Schadendorf D, Hassel JC, Eigentler TK, Martus P, Wolchok JD, Blank C, Pawelec G, Garbe C, Weide B (2016) Baseline peripheral blood biomarkers associated with clinical outcome of advanced melanoma patients treated with ipilimumab. Clin Cancer Res 22 (12):2908–2918. https://doi.org/10.1158/1078-0432.CCR-15-2412
2. Huang A, Zhang B, Wang B, Zhang F, Fan KX, Guo YJ (2013) Increased CD14(+)HLA-DR (-/low) myeloid-derived suppressor cells

correlate with extrathoracic metastasis and poor response to chemotherapy in non-small cell lung cancer patients. Cancer Immunol Immunother 62(9):1439–1451. https://doi.org/10.1007/s00262-013-1450-6

3. Santegoets SJ, Stam AG, Lougheed SM, Gall H, Jooss K, Sacks N, Hege K, Lowy I, Scheper RJ, Gerritsen WR, van den Eertwegh AJ, de Gruijl TD (2014) Myeloid derived suppressor and dendritic cell subsets are related to clinical outcome in prostate cancer patients treated with prostate GVAX and ipilimumab. J Immunother Cancer 2:31. https://doi.org/10.1186/s40425-014-0031-3
4. Walter S, Weinschenk T, Stenzl A, Zdrojowy R, Pluzanska A, Szczylik C, Staehler M, Brugger W, Dietrich PY, Mendrzyk R, Hilf N, Schoor O, Fritsche J, Mahr A, Maurer D, Vass V, Trautwein C, Lewandrowski P, Flohr C, Pohla H, Stanczak JJ, Bronte V, Mandruzzato S, Biedermann T, Pawelec G, Derhovanessian E, Yamagishi H, Miki T, Hongo F, Takaha N, Hirakawa K, Tanaka H, Stevanovic S, Frisch J, Mayer-Mokler A, Kirner A, Rammensee HG, Reinhardt C, Singh-Jasuja H (2012) Multipeptide immune response to cancer vaccine IMA901 after single-dose cyclophosphamide associates with longer patient survival. Nat Med 18 (8):1254–1261. https://doi.org/10.1038/nm.2883
5. Shipp C, Speigl L, Janssen N, Martens A, Pawelec G (2016) A clinical and biological perspective of human myeloid-derived suppressor cells in cancer. Cell Mol Life Sci 73 (21):4043–4061. https://doi.org/10.1007/s00018-016-2278-y
6. Sahin U, Derhovanessian E, Miller M, Kloke BP, Simon P, Lower M, Bukur V, Tadmor AD, Luxemburger U, Schrors B, Omokoko T, Vormehr M, Albrecht C, Paruzynski A, Kuhn AN, Buck J, Heesch S, Schreeb KH, Muller F, Ortseifer I, Vogler I, Godehardt E, Attig S, Rae R, Breitkreuz A, Tolliver C, Suchan M, Martic G, Hohberger A, Sorn P, Diekmann J, Ciesla J, Waksmann O, Bruck AK, Witt M, Zillgen M, Rothermel A, Kasemann B, Langer D, Bolte S, Diken M, Kreiter S, Nemecek R, Gebhardt C, Grabbe S, Holler C, Utikal J, Huber C, Loquai C, Tureci O (2017) Personalized RNA mutanome vaccines mobilize poly-specific therapeutic immunity against cancer. Nature 547(7662):222–226. https://doi.org/10.1038/nature23003
7. Weide B, Zelba H, Derhovanessian E, Pflugfelder A, Eigentler TK, Di Giacomo AM, Maio M, Aarntzen EH, de Vries IJ, Sucker A, Schadendorf D, Buttner P, Garbe C, Pawelec G (2012) Functional T cells targeting NY-ESO-1 or Melan-A are predictive for survival of patients with distant melanoma metastasis. J Clin Oncol 30(15):1835–1841. https://doi.org/10.1200/JCO.2011.40.2271
8. Rizvi NA, Hellmann MD, Snyder A, Kvistborg P, Makarov V, Havel JJ, Lee W, Yuan J, Wong P, Ho TS, Miller ML, Rekhtman N, Moreira AL, Ibrahim F, Bruggeman C, Gasmi B, Zappasodi R, Maeda Y, Sander C, Garon EB, Merghoub T, Wolchok JD, Schumacher TN, Chan TA (2015) Cancer immunology. Mutational landscape determines sensitivity to PD-1 blockade in non-small cell lung cancer. Science 348 (6230):124–128. https://doi.org/10.1126/science.aaa1348
9. Bacher P, Scheffold A (2013) Flow-cytometric analysis of rare antigen-specific T cells. Cytometry A 83(8):692–701. https://doi.org/10.1002/cyto.a.22317
10. Bailur JK, Gueckel B, Derhovanessian E, Pawelec G (2015) Presence of circulating Her2-reactive CD8 + T-cells is associated with lower frequencies of myeloid-derived suppressor cells and regulatory T cells, and better survival in older breast cancer patients. Breast Cancer Res 17:34. https://doi.org/10.1186/s13058-015-0541-z
11. Weide B, Martens A, Zelba H, Stutz C, Derhovanessian E, Di Giacomo AM, Maio M, Sucker A, Schilling B, Schadendorf D, Buttner P, Garbe C, Pawelec G (2014) Myeloid-derived suppressor cells predict survival of patients with advanced melanoma: comparison with regulatory T cells and NY-ESO-1- or melan-A-specific T cells. Clin Cancer Res 20(6):1601–1609. https://doi.org/10.1158/1078-0432.CCR-13-2508
12. Janssen N, Fortis SP, Speigl L, Haritos C, Sotiriadou NN, Sofopoulos M, Arnogiannaki N, Stavropoulos-Giokas C, Dinou A, Perez S, Pawelec G, Baxevanis CN, Shipp C (2017) Peripheral T cell responses to tumour antigens are associated with molecular, immunogenetic and cellular features of breast cancer patients. Breast Cancer Res Treat 161(1):51–62. https://doi.org/10.1007/s10549-016-4037-z

Chapter 11

Assessing Canonical and Adaptive Natural Killer Cell Function in Suppression Assays In Vitro

Dhifaf Sarhan and Jeffrey S. Miller

Abstract

The in vitro culture system outlined in this chapter allows for standardized protocols to examine canonical and adaptive natural killer (NK) cell responses while interacting with immune suppressor cells such as regulatory T cells (Treg) and myeloid-derived suppressor cells (MDSC). These interactions pathologically occur during tumorigenesis and tumor progression. Strategies to study the effects of ex vivo purified immune suppressor cells from cancer patients on the function of NK cell antitumor activity will help to understand suppressive mechanisms to improve immunotherapy. Immune checkpoint inhibitors have recently demonstrated tremendous clinical responses in patients with diverse types of cancers. However, their effect on NK cell function is not very well studied. Here, we have adapted a coculture system that previously has been utilized to study regulatory T cells. This approach can further be utilized to study the effects of immune checkpoint inhibitors in vitro and ex vivo. We focus on the differences between canonical NK cells and the newly identified subset of NK cells termed "adaptive NK cells." These cells are induced by cytomegalovirus (CMV) in CMV-seropositive individuals.

Key words Human canonical and adaptive NK cells, Immune suppression, Treg, MDSC

1 Introduction

Natural killer cells represent 5–15% of peripheral blood mononuclear cells [1]. They recognize and kill malignantly transformed and virally infected cells through an array of surface-expressed activating and inhibitory receptors. In addition, NK cells control the innate and the adaptive immune response in disease by secreting immune modulatory cytokines [2–4]. Although NK cells are expected to target malignantly transformed cells and play an important role in the immune surveillance against tumors, there is growing evidence suggesting that non-tumor cells within the tumor microenvironment negatively orchestrate the efficacy of cellular immunotherapy including regulatory T cells (Treg), myeloid-derived suppressor

Yago Pico de Coaña (ed.), *Immune Checkpoint Blockade: Methods and Protocols*, Methods in Molecular Biology, vol. 1913, https://doi.org/10.1007/978-1-4939-8979-9_11, © Springer Science+Business Media, LLC, part of Springer Nature 2019

cells (MDSC), cancer-associated fibroblasts (CAF), and tumor-associated macrophages (TAMs) [5]. It is now appreciated that changes in the NK cell receptor repertoire and ligand expression at the sites of primary tumor or metastases might result in decreased NK cell activity and thus lead to increased invasion and metastasis of tumors [6]. Such immune suppression could be mediated by increased expression of immune checkpoint proteins on tumor cells such as PD-1 and TIGIT [7, 8]. However, it is more likely that suppression is mediated by the interaction with immune suppressive cells that are found in the tumor microenvironment including Treg, MDSC, and TAM [9].

For decades, NK cells were described as innate immune cells that are unable to generate memory. However, recent groundbreaking research revealed that NK cells are capable of generating immunological memory against virus [10–12]. CMV exposure has profound effects on NK cell phenotype, proliferation, and function. A number of studies suggest that NK cells can develop immunological memory against viral exposure such as CMV and nonviral haptens [13, 14]. These cells persist long-term in vivo, demonstrate augmented function following a secondary stimulation, and undergo several classical memory phases: expansion, contraction, and memory [13, 15]. We have identified heterogeneous subsets of highly specialized human NK cells that arise in response to CMV infection. These cells are referred to as "adaptive," and they are characterized by a common epigenetic downregulation of the transcription factor PLZF and additional proximal signaling molecules SYK, EAT-2, and FcεR1γ. These adaptive NK cells express NKG2C and CD57 and exhibit elevated cytokine production induced by CD16 ligation [12]. However, the physiologic role of this newly discovered subpopulation of NK cells especially the contribution to the immune surveillance against tumors is still unknown. Bryceson et al. reported that adaptive NK cells persist in individuals with *GATA2* mutation, where canonical NK cells are lost [16]. *GATA2* encodes the GATA-2 protein, which is a transcription factor required for hematopoietic stem and progenitor cell (HSPC) survival and proliferation [17]. On the other hand, mutations in *SAMD9L*, a tumor suppressor gene, might affect adaptive NK cell development [18]. These findings suggest that canonical and adaptive NK cell development depends on different transcription factors. Recent discoveries have been made by our laboratory to understand adaptive NK cells in the tumor microenvironment. We found that adaptive NK cells have a distinct receptor repertoire compared to canonical NK cells that results in unique resistance to Treg (unpublished data) and MDSC suppression [19]. Moreover, in another study we have shown that adaptive NK cell expansion is associated with reduced leukemia relapse [20]. Thus, adaptive NK cells have therapeutic potential for cancer cell therapies. Therefore, a standardized protocol to study this subpopulation in vitro is needed.

NK cell function in vitro has commonly been assessed by a short-term (4 h) 51-Cr release assay against the NK cell-sensitive cell line K562 [21]. The advantage of using K562 as a target for testing NK cell function is the lack of major histocompatibility complex class I (MHCI) expression needed for non-self-recognition and the ability to test function within the mononuclear cell (MNC) population without further separation [22]. However, using tumor cells alone does not represent the tumor microenvironment. Therefore, adding immune suppressor cells to the tumor and NK cell coculture might give a more precise measure of the complexity of the tumor microenvironment. A protocol to study the interaction between NK cell different subsets and immune suppressor cells is outlined here.

2 Materials

This protocol includes the experimental procedures that our laboratory has developed to examine adaptive and canonical NK cell function in a 5–6-day-long culture in order to study the effects of immune suppressor cells.

2.1 CMV+ Donors and NK Cell Isolation

If possible, experiments should start with CMV-seropositive blood donors, containing a population of adaptive NK cells. If that is not possible, adaptive NK cell numbers, defined as $CD56^{+}CD3^{-}CD57^{+}NKG2C^{+}$ (Fig. 1), should be determined before coculture and will define the adaptive NK cell population. It is best to start these experiments with >5% of these cells.

1. CMV-seropositive donors.
2. Ficoll-Paque Plus.
3. ACK lysing buffer.
4. PBS/0.5% AB human serum/2 mM EDTA.
5. EasySep™ human NK cell enrichment kit (StemCell Technologies).
6. Peripheral blood mononuclear cells from CMV^{+} donors.
7. EasyEights™ EasySep™ magnet (StemCell Technologies).

2.2 HLA-DR+ Cell Isolation

Allogeneic $HLA\text{-}DR^{+}$ antigen-presenting cells (APCs) are utilized instead of anti-CD3/CD28 stimulation beads in this protocol to avoid artificial stimulation of Treg.

1. Peripheral blood mononuclear cells (PBMC) from CMV^{+} donors.
2. EasyEights™ EasySep™ magnet (StemCell Technologies).

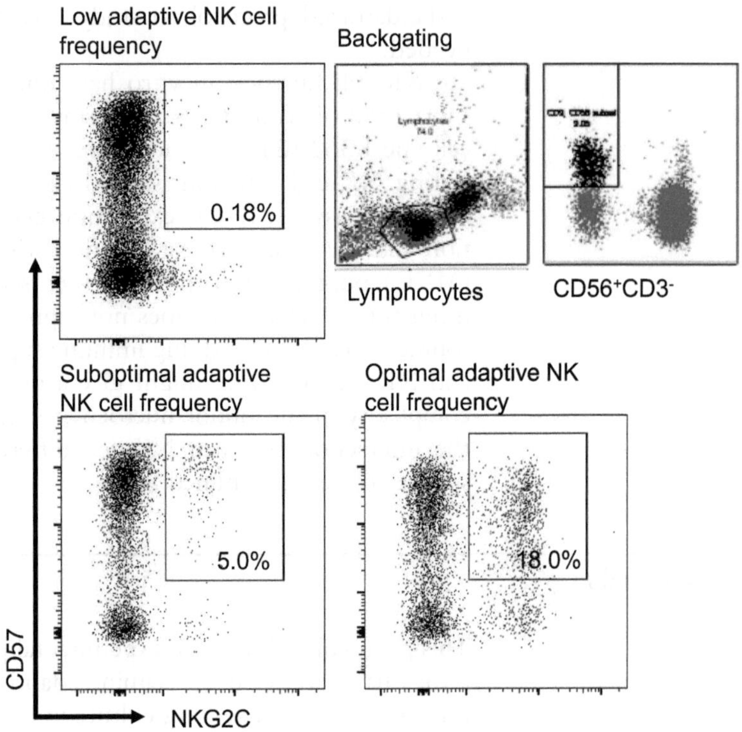

Fig. 1 PBMC from CMV-seropositive blood donors were stained for CD56, CD3, CD56, CD57, and NKG2C for determination of bulk adaptive NK cell frequencies of total NK cells following ficoll separation

3. Anti-HLA-DR MicroBeads (Miltenyi Biotech).
4. MACS® MS separation columns (Miltenyi Biotech).
5. MACS® pre-separation filters (Miltenyi Biotech).
6. MACS® magnetic stand and magnets (Miltenyi Biotech).

2.3 MDSC In Vitro Generation

MDSC accumulation is a prognostic factor in many cancer types. Generation of MDSC in vitro allowed for discoveries of immune suppression mechanisms in cancer. We have previously reported that MDSC from patients with melanoma suppress canonical NK cells through mechanisms involving tumor-derived prostaglandin-e2 that induced elevated secretion of TGFβ in MDSC [23]. However, later we discovered that adaptive NK cells are resistant to MDSC suppression as a result of low expression of TIGIT [19]. Here we use a protocol to generate highly suppressive MDSC that resemble MDSC characteristics in vivo [24].

1. CD33 MicroBeads (Miltenyi Biotech).
2. MACS® LS and MS separation columns (Miltenyi Biotech).
3. MACS® pre-separation filters (Miltenyi Biotech).

4. MACS® magnetic stand and magnets (Miltenyi Biotech).
5. GM-CSF (R&D Systems).
6. IL-6 (Sigma-Aldrich).
7. 6-well cell culture plates.

2.4 Treg

Tumor progression promotes the recruitment and generation of intratumoral Treg, associated with a poor prognosis in cancer patients. To target the suppressive network of the tumor microenvironment, we need to better understand the interplay between Treg and immune effector cells. Here, we are using expanded natural Treg. If users wish to expand own Treg, follow the protocols described in the following references [25, 26].

1. IL-2.
2. X-vivo 15 cell culture medium (Lonza).
3. T75 (75 cm^2) cell culture flasks.

2.5 Medium and Reagents

All media are prepared freshly and serums are heat inactivated.

1. Basal medium: RPMI and 10% fetal bovine serum (FBS).
2. MDSC culture medium: RPBMI, 10% fetal bovine serum (FBS) supplemented with final concentrations of IL-10 (10 ng/mL) and IL-6 (10 ng/mL).
3. Treg: X-vivo 15, 10% AB human serum and IL-2 (300 IU/mL).
4. NK cell cytokines: IL-2 (50 IU/mL) or IL-15 (10 ng/mL).
5. Freezing medium: 10% Dimetylsulfoxid (DMSO) in FBS.
6. Blocking antibodies against PD-1 (10 μg/mL) and TIGIT (10 μg/mL).

2.6 FACS-Based Functional Assay and Staining

1. Agonistic anti-CD16 (Biolegend).
2. IL-18 (50 ng/mL).
3. IL-12 (5 ng/mL).
4. Foxp3/transcription factor fixation and permeabilization kit (eBioscience).
5. Fluorescence-conjugated antibodies:

Marker	Clone	Fluorochrome	Manufactory
CD3	OKT3	BV785	Biolegend
CD56	NCAM	PE/CY7	Biolegend
CD57	NK-1	BV605	BD biosciences
NKG2C	134,591	PE	R&D systems

(continued)

Marker	Clone	Fluorochrome	Manufactory
FCεRγ	RB polyclonal	FITC	EMD millipore
CD107a	H4A3	PerCP/Cy5.5	Biolegend
IFNγ	4S.B3	BV650	Biolegend
Ki67	B56	AF700	BD biosciences
Fixable dead cell marker		Near-IR	Invitrogen

6. LSRII or Fortessa (Becton Dickinson) for acquisition of data and FlowJo 10.0 for analyzing of data

3 Methods

3.1 Day 0 MDSC Generation and Determination of Adaptive NK Cell Numbers

1. Transfer blood into a sterile container, and dilute blood with PBS/0.5% AB human serum/2 mM EDTA 1:1 from buffy coat (40 mL) or 1:5 from trima cones (10 mL).
2. Prepare 50 Falcone tubes (2–3 per donor) with 15–20 mL Ficoll-Paque Plus.
3. Slowly and carefully lay the diluted blood on the ficoll (25–30 mL/tube).
4. Centrifuge at 750 × *g* for 20 min at room temperature with low acceleration and brake off.
5. Slowly harvest the lymphocyte interface (white band), and transfer to a new 50 mL centrifuge tube. Fill up to 50 mL with buffer and centrifuge at 500 × *g* for 10 min.
6. Gently decant the supernatant and resuspend cells in 40 mL cold buffer and centrifuge at 200 × *g* for 8 min.
7. Add 5 mL ACK lysing buffer per donor to lysate the remaining red blood cells if necessary and incubate for 3 min in RT.
8. Fill up to 40 mL with buffer and centrifuge at 500 × *g* for 10 min.
9. Determine total cell number using a Countess® automated cell counter.
10. Stain a sample of cells for CD56, CD3, CD57, and NKG2C to determine the frequency of bulk adaptive NK cells (Fig. 1 *for gating strategy*). Less than 5% might be insufficient to be informative for adaptive NK cells.
11. Label cells (1×10^8) from CMV+ donors with optimal adaptive NK cell subpopulation for isolation of CD33+ cells to generate MDSC by adding 100 μL CD33 (*see* **Note 1**) microbeads and 400 μL PBS/0.5% AB human serum/2 mM

EDTA for every 10^8 cells. Incubate for 15 min on ice in the dark or in the fridge.

12. While waiting, set up one MACS® LS column per blood donor on a MACS® magnetic stand. Place a MACS® pre-separation filter on top of each column, and wash the column with 3 mL of buffer.
13. Add 20 mL of PBS/0.5% AB human serum/2 mM EDTA to the cells, and centrifuge for 5 min at 500 × *g*.
14. Gently discard the supernatant and resuspend the cells in 0.5 mL buffer.
15. Pipette the labeled cells into a pre-separation filter, and let the cells pass through the column. There is no need to save the effluent, as the CD33+ cells will be retained within the column.
16. Wash the column three times with buffer (3 mL × 3).
17. Remove the pre-separation filter, pull the column off the magnet, and transfer the column to a 15-mL centrifuge tube. Apply 5 mL of buffer and forcefully plunge the liquid through the column to collect the labeled cells.
18. Count the total number of cells and centrifuge cells for 5 min at 500 × *g*.
19. Gently decant the supernatant, and resuspend the cell pellet in MDSC medium at a concentration of 2 × 10^6 cells/mL. Transfer the cells in into a 6-well 2 mL/well and place in an incubator set to 37 °C 5% CO2. The number of cells isolated will vary between blood donors but typically will get 10–15% CD33+ cells.
20. Freeze down the rest of the PBMC for later isolation of monocytes and NK cells at a concentration of 1 × 10^8 per tube in freezing medium.

3.2 Day 3 or 4 Maintenance of MDSC

1. Add 1 mL per well fresh pre-warmed (37 °C water bath) MDSC medium with additional cytokines to a final concentration of 10 ng/mL of IL-16 and IL-10.
2. Incubate for another 3–4 days.

3.3 Day 6 Recovery of PBMC and Treg from Cryopreservation

1. Thaw PBMC (*see* **Note 2**) from autologous donors to MDSC by adding cells to 10 mL RT pre-warmed medium.
2. Centrifuge cells for 5 min at 500 × *g*.
3. Discard supernatant and resuspend cells in 10 mL medium.
4. Count cells.
5. Centrifuge cells for 5 min at 500 × *g*.
6. Resuspend cells in 37 °C pre-warmed RPMI + 10% FBS medium at concentration of 4–5 M cells/mL, and culture in T75 flask horizontally in 37 °C 5% CO_2 incubator overnight.

7. Thaw allogeneic Treg (*see* **Note 3**) by repeating **steps 24–27**.
8. Resuspend cells in Treg medium at a concentration of 0.5–1 M/mL, and culture in T75 flask horizontally in 37 °C 5% CO_2 incubator overnight.

3.4 Day 7 Isolation of NK Cells and Accessory Cells

1. Collect overnight rested PBMC from flasks and spin down at 500 × *g* for 5 min.
2. Discard supernatant and resuspend cells in 20 mL buffer.
3. Take 10 μL of sample and dilute 1:10 in PBS in a counting plate and count cells by Countess® automated cell counter.
4. Allocate 20 million MNC cells each for APC and CD33 (control for MDSC) cell isolation and the rest of PBMC for NK cell isolation.
5. Isolate APC or CD33 cells by labeling 2×10^7 cells with 20 μL HLA-DR$^+$ or CD33 microbeads (*see* **Note 1**) and 80 μL PBS/0.5% AB human serum/2 mM EDTA. Incubate for 15 min on ice in the dark or in the fridge.
6. While waiting, set up one MACS® MS column per blood donor on a MACS® magnetic stand. Place a MACS® pre-separation filter on top of each column, and wash the column with 2 mL of buffer.
7. Add 4 mL of PBS/0.5% AB human serum/2 mM EDTA to the cells, and centrifuge for 5 min at 500 × *g*.
8. Gently discard the supernatant and resuspend the cells in 0.5 mL buffer.
9. Pipette the labeled cells into pre-separation filter and let the cells pass through the column. There is no need to save the effluent, as the CD33+ and HLA-DR+ cells will be retained within the column.
10. Wash the column three times with 0.5 mL buffer.
11. Remove the pre-separation filter, pull the column off the magnet, and transfer the column to a 15-mL centrifuge tube. Apply 2 mL of buffer, and forcefully plunge the liquid through the column to collect the labeled cells.
12. Count the total cell number and centrifuge cells for 5 min at 500 × *g*.
13. Gently decant the supernatant, and resuspend the cell pellet in NK cells medium at a concentration of 1×10^6 cells/mL.
14. Next isolate NK cells by negative depletion. Resuspend 5×10^7 in 1 mL buffer and label with 50 μL of enrichment cocktail in 10 min in RT.
15. Vortex magnetic particles for 30 s before use.

16. Add magnetic particles 100 μL/mL of sample and incubate for 5 min in RT.
17. Fill up to 3 mL or to 7 mL depending on the sample size by either using 5 mL or 10 mL polystyrene round-bottom tubes.
18. Place sample tubes into the magnets and incubate for 2.5 min.
19. Pick up the magnet, and in one motion invert the magnet with the tube (s), and pour off the enriched NK cell suspension into a new tube (s).
20. Count cells and spin for 5 min.
21. Resuspend the cell pellet at a concentration of 1×10^6 cells/mL in basal medium.

3.5 Coculture of NK Cells and Immune Suppressive Cells

1. Add 100 μL NK cells (*see* **Notes 4** and **5**) and 100 μL MDSC that give 1:1 ratio per well in u-bottom 96-well plate ± anti-TIGIT (10 μg/mL), anti-PD-1 (10 μg/mL), or appropriate isotype control.
2. Alternatively, add 50 μL NK cells and 50 μL APC that give 1:1 ratio with or without 25 μL Treg that give 1:2 ratio per well in u-bottom 96-well plate ± anti-TIGIT (10 μg/mL), anti-PD-1 (10 μg/mL), or appropriate isotype control.
3. Top up all wells to 200 μL/well supplemented with a final concentration of 10 ng/mL IL-15 for NK-MDSC coculture and 50 IU/mL IL-2 for NK-Treg coculture.
4. Place plates in an incubator set to 37 °C and 5% CO_2 and incubate for 5–6 days.

3.6 Stimulation and Analysis

Following 5 or 6 days of coculture with immune suppressor cells, NK cells are stimulated with agonistic CD16 and IL-18 and IL-12 for 6 h prior to analysis (*see* **Note 6**). We perform a FACS-based analysis to measure NK cell degranulation by surface CD107a expression and intracellular IFN-γ production.

3.6.1 On Day 5 for NK Cell-MDSC and Day 6 for NK Cell-Treg Cocultures

1. Add 30 μL RP10 medium alone or supplemented with agonistic anti-CD16 (1 μg/mL) IL-12 (5 ng/mL) and IL-18 (50 ng/mL) (*see* **Note 6**).
2. Add 2 μL CD107a PerCP-Cy5.5 and GolgiPlug (1: 1000) and GolgiStop (1:1000) to all wells.
3. Incubate at 37 °C for 4–6 h.
4. Spin down at 750 × *g* for 2 min, and decant supernatant.
5. Add 50 μL of surface antibodies in PBS and live/dead dye (0.2 μL/well) to each well.
6. Incubate at 4 °C for 20 min.
7. Add 150 μL buffer and spin down at 750 × *g* for 2 min, and discard supernatant.

8. Add 200 μL buffer, spin down at 750 × *g* for 2 min, and discard supernatant.
9. Add 80 μL 1× fix/perm buffer.
10. Incubate at RT for 20 min (dark).
11. Add 150 μL perm wash.
12. Spin down at 750 × *g* for 2 min, and discard supernatant.
13. Add 50 μL intracellular antibody cocktail including IFNγ, TNFα, and FcεRγ (*see* **Note** 7).
14. Incubate at RT for 35 min (dark).
15. Add 150 μL perm wash.
16. Spin down at 750 × *g* for 2 min, and discard supernatant.
17. Wash with 200 μL buffer.
18. Add 200 μL of buffer.
19. Transfer to small flow tubes "bullets."
20. Keep samples on ice before and during run.
21. Run by FACS LSRII or Fortessa (Becton Dickinson).
22. Analyze data by FlowJo (Figs. 2 and 3).

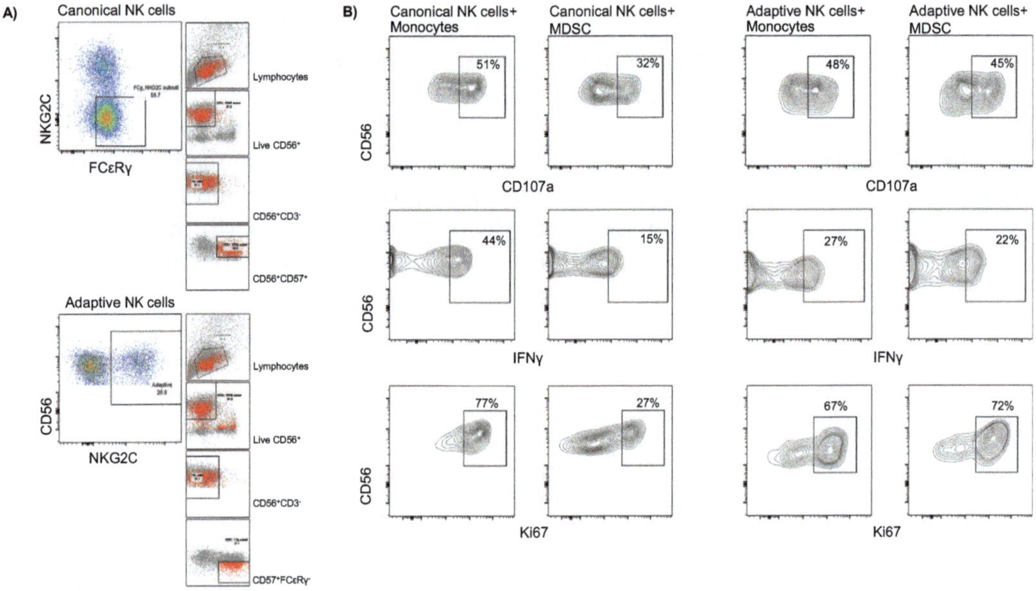

Fig. 2 Purified NK cells were cocultured with monocytes or MDSCs at a 1:1 ratio in the presence of IL-15 (10 ng/mL) for 5 days. Cells were stimulated with agonistic CD16 (1 μg/mL) for 6 h prior to staining and evaluated for degranulation (CD107a), IFN-γ production, and proliferation (Ki67). Representative data are shown for (**a**) canonical and adaptive NK cell gating and (**b**) NK cell function

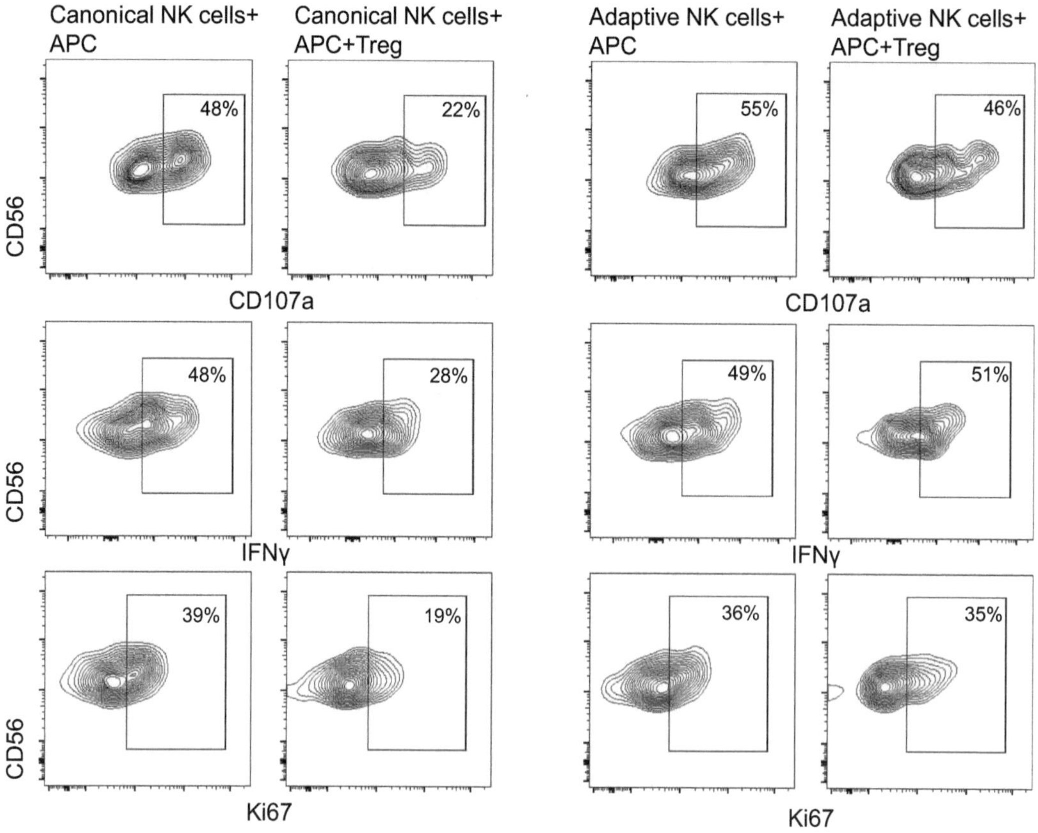

Fig. 3 Purified NK cells were cocultured with APC ± Treg for 6 days in the presence of IL-2 (50 IU/mL) and stimulated with anti-CD16, IL-12, and IL-18 6 h prior to analysis. Representative data are shown

4 Notes

Following optimization in our laboratory, we suggest the following recommendations:

1. The amount of microbeads used in the isolation protocols are optimized in our lab, and therefore, we use half of the microbead amount that is recommended by the manufacturer.
2. Ca. 20–30% of cells are lost following freezing; therefore, we usually thaw two to three vials of cryopreserved PBMC for sufficient NK cell numbers after isolation.
3. There is considerable variety in the capacity of suppression of MDSC and Treg from different donors; therefore, three or more donors are recommended to include within the individual experiments.
4. NK cell numbers per well in a 96-well plate shouldn't be less than 3×10^4 and more than 1×10^5 for optimal cell clustering

and proliferation. Too few NK cells will not build clusters, and too many cells will suffer from lack of space.

5. Experimental duplicates or triplicates are included and pooled prior to staining for sufficient cell numbers for analysis.
6. Adaptive NK cells are less responsive to IL-12 and IL-18 stimulation, likely due to low IL-12/IL-18 receptor expression, but they are more sensitive to stimulation by CD16 ligation compared to canonical NK cells [12]. Therefore, to stimulate both canonical and adaptive NK cells equally, the agonistic anti-CD16 antibody in addition to IL-12/IL-18 is used to study function.
7. Bulk adaptive NK cells are identified as $CD56^+CD57^+NKG2C^+$; however, there are small subpopulations within those cells that downregulate PLZF, Syk, and/or FcεR1γ that could be separately analyzed. In this protocol we have focused on FcεR1γ subpopulation as they achieve better resistance to immune suppressive cells.

Acknowledgments

This work was funded in part with federal funds from the National Cancer Institute (NCI), NIH, CA111412, and CA65493.

References

1. Caligiuri MA (2008) Human natural killer cells. Blood 112(3):461–469. https://doi.org/10.1182/blood-2007-09-077438
2. Lanier LL (2008) Up on the tightrope: natural killer cell activation and inhibition. Nat Immunol 9(5):495–502. https://doi.org/10.1038/ni1581
3. Vivier E, Tomasello E, Baratin M, Walzer T, Ugolini S (2008) Functions of natural killer cells. Nat Immunol 9(5):503–510. https://doi.org/10.1038/ni1582
4. Raulet DH (2004) Interplay of natural killer cells and their receptors with the adaptive immune response. Nat Immunol 5(10):996–1002. https://doi.org/10.1038/ni1114
5. Vitale M, Cantoni C, Pietra G, Mingari MC, Moretta L (2014) Effect of tumor cells and tumor microenvironment on NK-cell function. Eur J Immunol 44(6):1582–1592. https://doi.org/10.1002/eji.201344272
6. Lopez-Soto A, Gonzalez S, Smyth MJ, Galluzzi L (2017) Control of metastasis by NK cells. Cancer Cell 32(2):135–154. https://doi.org/10.1016/j.ccell.2017.06.009
7. Benson DM Jr, Bakan CE, Mishra A, Hofmeister CC, Efebera Y, Becknell B, Baiocchi RA, Zhang J, Yu J, Smith MK, Greenfield CN, Porcu P, Devine SM, Rotem-Yehudar R, Lozanski G, Byrd JC, Caligiuri MA (2010) The PD-1/PD-L1 axis modulates the natural killer cell versus multiple myeloma effect: a therapeutic target for CT-011, a novel monoclonal anti-PD-1 antibody. Blood 116(13):2286–2294. https://doi.org/10.1182/blood-2010-02-271874
8. Stanietsky N, Simic H, Arapovic J, Toporik A, Levy O, Novik A, Levine Z, Beiman M, Dassa L, Achdout H, Stern-Ginossar N, Tsukerman P, Jonjic S, Mandelboim O (2009) The interaction of TIGIT with PVR and PVRL2 inhibits human NK cell cytotoxicity. Proc Natl Acad Sci U S A 106(42):17858–17863. https://doi.org/10.1073/pnas.0903474106
9. Hasmim M, Messai Y, Ziani L, Thiery J, Bouhris JH, Noman MZ, Chouaib S (2015) Critical role of tumor microenvironment in shaping NK cell functions: implication of hypoxic

stress. Front Immunol 6. https://doi.org/10.3389/fimmu.2015.00482

10. O'Sullivan TE, Sun JC (2015) Generation of natural killer cell memory during viral infection. J Innate Immun 7(6):557–562. https://doi.org/10.1159/000375494
11. Lopez-Verges S, Milush JM, Schwartz BS, Pando MJ, Jarjoura J, York VA, Houchins JP, Miller S, Kang SM, Norris PJ, Nixon DF, Lanier LL (2011) Expansion of a unique CD57(+)NKG2Chi natural killer cell subset during acute human cytomegalovirus infection. Proc Natl Acad Sci U S A 108 (36):14725–14732. https://doi.org/10.1073/pnas.1110900108
12. Schlums H, Cichocki F, Tesi B, Theorell J, Beziat V, Holmes TD, Han H, Chiang SC, Foley B, Mattsson K, Larsson S, Schaffer M, Malmberg KJ, Ljunggren HG, Miller JS, Bryceson YT (2015) Cytomegalovirus infection drives adaptive epigenetic diversification of NK cells with altered signaling and effector function. Immunity 42(3):443–456. https://doi.org/10.1016/j.immuni.2015.02.008
13. Sun JC, Beilke JN, Lanier LL (2009) Adaptive immune features of natural killer cells. Nature 457(7229):557–561. https://doi.org/10.1038/nature07665
14. Paust S, Gill HS, Wang BZ, Flynn MP, Moseman EA, Senman B, Szczepanik M, Telenti A, Askenase PW, Compans RW, von Andrian UH (2010) Critical role for the chemokine receptor CXCR6 in NK cell-mediated antigen-specific memory of haptens and viruses. Nat Immunol 11(12):1127–1135. https://doi.org/10.1038/ni.1953
15. O'Sullivan TE, Sun JC, Lanier LL (2015) Natural killer cell memory. Immunity 43 (4):634–645. https://doi.org/10.1016/j.immuni.2015.09.013
16. Schlums H, Jung M, Han HY, Theorell J, Bigley V, Chiang SCC, Allan DSJ, Davidson-Moncada JK, Dickinson RE, Holmes TD, Hsu AP, Townsley D, Winkler T, Wang WX, Aukrust P, Nordoy I, Calvo KR, Holland SM, Collin M, Dunbar CE, Bryceson YT (2017) Adaptive NK cells can persist in patients with GATA2 mutation depleted of stem and progenitor cells. Blood 129(14):1927–1939. https://doi.org/10.1182/blood-2016-08734236
17. Tsai FY, Keller G, Kuo FC, Weiss M, Chen J, Rosenblatt M, Alt FW, Orkin SH (1994) An early haematopoietic defect in mice lacking the transcription factor GATA-2. Nature 371 (6494):221–226. https://doi.org/10.1038/371221a0
18. Tesi B, Davidsson J, Voss M, Rahikkala E, Holmes TD, Chiang SCC, Komulainen-Ebrahim J, Gorcenco S, Rundberg Nilsson A, Ripperger T, Kokkonen H, Bryder D, Fioretos T, Henter JI, Mottonen M, Niinimaki R, Nilsson L, Pronk CJ, Puschmann A, Qian H, Uusimaa J, Moilanen J, Tedgard U, Cammenga J, Bryceson YT (2017) Gain-of-function SAMD9L mutations cause a syndrome of cytopenia, immunodeficiency, MDS, and neurological symptoms. Blood 129(16):2266–2279. https://doi.org/10.1182/blood-2016-10-743302
19. Sarhan D, Cichocki F, Zhang B, Yingst A, Spellman SR, Cooley S, Verneris MR, Blazar BR, Miller JS (2016) Adaptive NK cells with low TIGIT expression are inherently resistant to myeloid-derived suppressor cells. Cancer Res 76(19):5696–5706. https://doi.org/10.1158/0008-5472.CAN-16-0839
20. Cichocki F, Cooley S, Davis Z, DeFor TE, Schlums H, Zhang B, Brunstein CG, Blazar BR, Wagner J, Diamond DJ, Verneris MR, Bryceson YT, Weisdorf DJ, Miller JS (2016) CD56dimCD57+NKG2C+ NK cell expansion is associated with reduced leukemia relapse after reduced intensity HCT. Leukemia 30 (2):456–463. https://doi.org/10.1038/leu.2015.260
21. Nagel JE, Collins GD, Adler WH (1981) Spontaneous or natural-killer cyto-toxicity of K562 erythroleukemic cells in normal-patients. Cancer Res 41(6):2284–2288
22. Brunner KT, Mauel J, Cerottini JC, Chapuis B (1968) Quantitative assay of lytic action of immune lymphoid cells on 51cr-labelled allogeneic target cells in vitro—inhibition by isoantibody and by drugs. Immunology 14 (2):181–196
23. Mao Y, Sarhan D, Steven A, Seliger B, Kiessling R, Lundqvist A (2014) Inhibition of tumor-derived prostaglandin-e2 blocks the induction of myeloid-derived suppressor cells and recovers natural killer cell activity. Clin Cancer Res 20(15):4096–4106. https://doi.org/10.1158/1078-0432.CCR-14-0635
24. Lechner MG, Liebertz DJ, Epstein AL (2010) Characterization of cytokine-induced myeloid-derived suppressor cells from normal human peripheral blood mononuclear cells. J Immunol 185(4):2273–2284. https://doi.org/10.4049/jimmunol.1000901
25. Hippen KL, Merkel SC, Schirm DK, Nelson C, Tennis NC, Riley JL, June CH, Miller JS, Wagner JE, Blazar BR (2011) Generation and large-scale expansion of human inducible

regulatory T cells that suppress graft-versus-host disease. Am J Transplant 11 (6):1148–1157. https://doi.org/10.1111/j.1600-6143.2011.03558.x

26. Hippen KL, Merkel SC, Schirm DK, Sieben CM, Sumstad D, Kadidlo DM, McKenna DH, Bromberg JS, Levine BL, Riley JL, June CH, Scheinberg P, Douek DC, Miller JS, Wagner JE, Blazar BR (2011) Massive ex vivo expansion of human natural regulatory T cells (T-regs) with minimal loss of in vivo functional activity. Sci Transl Med 3(83). https://doi.org/10.1126/scitranslmed.3001809

Chapter 12

Evaluating Antibody-Dependent Cell-Mediated Cytotoxicity by Chromium Release Assay

Irene van der Haar Àvila, Patricia Marmol, Rolf Kiessling, and Yago Pico de Coaña

Abstract

Antibody-dependent cell-mediated cytotoxicity (ADCC) is a mechanism in which immune cell activation is induced by the cross-linking of CD16 with the Fc region of antibodies that at the same time bind specifically to cell surface antigens. ADCC stimulates the secretion of perforin, granzymes, and cytokines leading to lysis of the malignant cells. Natural killer (NK) cells express the CD16 receptor and can therefore be activated by ADCC to kill tumor cells. To study the cytotoxicity of NK cells against cancer cells, an ADCC-based assay is described: the chromium release assay. In this method, the antibody trastuzumab, which binds specifically to HER2-positive malignant cells, is used to trigger ADCC.

Key words Antibody cell-mediated cytotoxicity, Natural killer cells, Trastuzumab, Chromium release assay

1 Introduction

Recently, there has been rapid progress in the field of clinical immunotherapy. In particular, the use of monoclonal antibodies (mAbs) for cancer therapy is one of the most effective strategies for treating cancer patients. Such mAbs can kill tumor cells by (1) blocking the function of the target molecule, (2) mediating the delivery of cytotoxic drugs, (3) affecting the tumor vasculature or stroma, and/or (4) triggering immune-mediated cell-killing mechanisms, such as antibody-dependent cell-mediated cytotoxicity (ADCC) [1]. ADCC occurs when the Fc-γ (CD16) receptor of effector immune cells becomes activated after interaction with antibodies. Natural killer (NK) cells, macrophages, and granulocytes express the CD16 receptor that recognizes the Fc region of IgG antibodies [2]. These antibodies can bind specifically to antigens that are expressed on malignant cells. At the same time, they can cross-link with the Fc receptors, triggering cell activation and

Yago Pico de Coaña (ed.), *Immune Checkpoint Blockade: Methods and Protocols*, Methods in Molecular Biology, vol. 1913, https://doi.org/10.1007/978-1-4939-8979-9_12, © Springer Science+Business Media, LLC, part of Springer Nature 2019

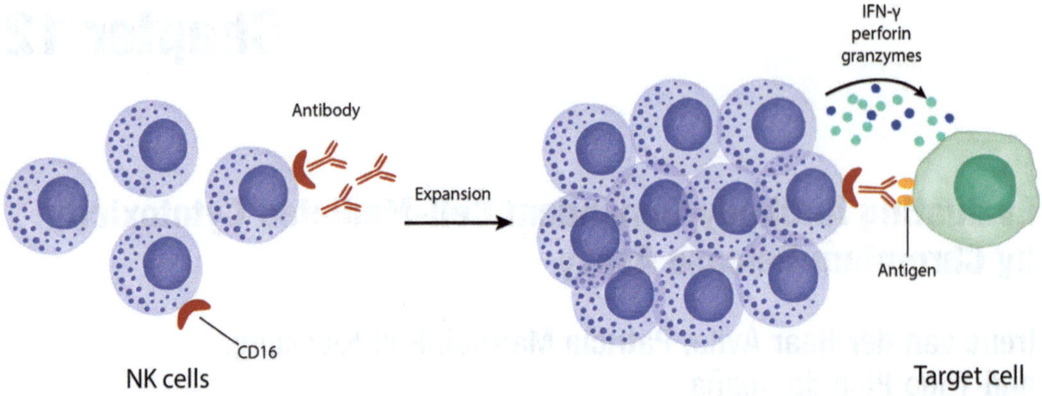

Fig. 1 Schematic representation of antibody-dependent cellular cytotoxicity (ADCC) mediated by NK cells. Using a specific antibody that binds to the CD16 Fc receptors and to tumor-associated antigens, NK cells become activated via antibody-dependent cell-mediated cytotoxicity inducing IFNγ, perforin, and granzymes release (Adapted from Morvan et al. [2])

secretion of cytokines such as IFNγ and granzymes, resulting in target cell lysis (Fig. 1) [3, 4].

There are already some clinically approved antibodies where ADCC has shown to participate as the active mechanism. One example is trastuzumab (Herceptin), a humanized mAb directed against the extracellular domain of the HER2 receptor [1]. Trastuzumab is widely used in the treatment of HER2-positive cancers, including breast cancer and ovarian cancer, among others [5, 6]. It binds to the CD16 receptor and to the HER2/neu receptor of malignant cells inducing immune-mediated responses.

The cytotoxicity of NK cells mediated by antibody immunotherapy can be studied by flow cytometry or by chromium (^{51}Cr) release assays. With flow cytometry, living and dead target and effector cells can be detected and quantified based on differential staining by fluorescent dyes [1]. CFSE (carboxyfluorescein succinimidyl ester) can be used as a dye to specifically label the target cell population to distinguish target and effector cells.

In ^{51}Cr release assays, the release of radioactive chromium from pre-labeled target cells is measured. The cells take up the radioisotope which then binds intracellularly to macromolecules. As long as the labeled cells are viable, the ^{51}Cr-macromolecule complexes remain contained in the cell because they cannot cross the membrane [7]. When the cells are lysed, the contents of the cell are released and therefore also the radioactive chromium, which can then be measured. This method has long been the most widely used technique for measuring cell-mediated cytotoxicity [1, 8] and was the first method used to evaluate ADCC [9]. The advantage of using chromium release assays is that less cells are needed and thus more conditions can be tested. However, it has some disadvantages, such as toxicity for target cells, low sensitivity, labeling

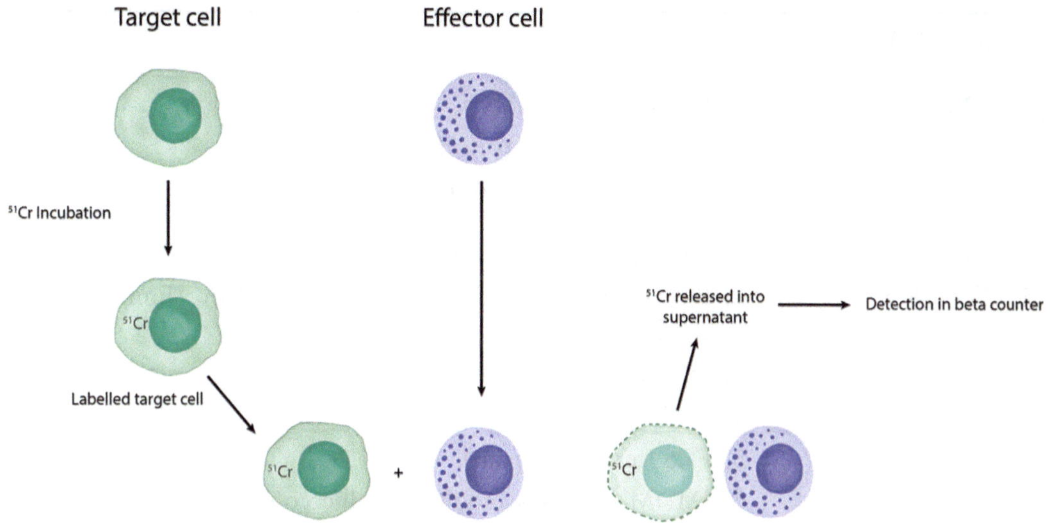

Fig. 2 Schematic overview of the chromium release assay. The procedure can be divided in three main steps: ^{51}Cr labeling of target cells, ^{51}Cr release by lysis, and detection of the released ^{51}Cr

irregularities, and the generation of radioactive waste [10]. In contrast, flow cytometry-based cytotoxicity assays are more sensitive and reproducible, and both live and dead populations of target and effector cells can be visualized. With this approach, it is also possible to perform immunophenotyping at the single-cell level. Since these cells are not cultured with toxic isotopes, long-term cultures can be maintained, and thus long-term effects on cytotoxicity can be studied [1]. However, for the flow cytometry assays, a higher number of cells are needed.

Here, we describe a ^{51}Cr release assay to evaluate ADCC in NK cells with the antibody trastuzumab. A brief overview of the chromium release method can be seen in Fig. 2. Target cells are labeled with ^{51}Cr and are then incubated with effector cells that are able to recognize and kill target cells by lysis. The supernatant containing the released chromium is collected and measured in a gamma counter or liquid scintillation counter, from which the cytotoxicity can be calculated.

^{51}Cr is a radioisotope that emits gamma rays and is thus hazardous to the health of people working with it. Therefore, some precautions should be taken such as working in special facilities, wearing protective gloves, and working in a special radioactive hood. It is produced in a reactor by neutron activation, and it decays by electron capture, emitting γ rays. Chromium has a half-life of 27.7 days. The principal gamma-photon emission occurs by electron capture at 320 keV. The high energy and low yield (9.8%) of gamma-photon emissions from decay of this radionuclide need a larger NaI crystal counter for efficient detection [11].

2 Materials

2.1 Cells

1. Fresh/frozen PBMCs.
2. Purified NK cells (or other effector cells).
3. Target cells (SkBr3 or other cell lines).

2.2 Reagents and Chemicals

1. 1 mCi/ml ^{51}chromium (Perkin Elmer, USA).
2. DC medium CellGro GMP + 2% HSA (human serum albumin).
3. DNase I recombinant (Roche, Germany).
4. 99.5% ethanol.
5. FCS (fetal calf serum).
6. IMDM (Iscove's modified Dulbecco's medium) + 10% FCS (fetal calf serum).
7. PBS (phosphate buffered saline).
8. RPMI 1640 (Roswell Park Memorial Institute) + 10% FCS (fetal calf serum) + penicillin/streptomycin.
9. 5% Triton X-100 (detergent) (Merck, Sweden) in RPMI medium.
10. Trypan blue.
11. 0.48 mM versene solution.

2.3 Antibodies and Cytokines

1. CD3-PO-conjugated antibody (Invitrogen, UK).
2. CD56-PE-Cy7-conjugated antibody (BioLegend, San Diego, USA).
3. 18×10^5 U/ml IL-2 (Novartis, Copenhagen, Denmark).
4. 5.3 mg/ml isotype control, hIgG1 (BMS, NY, USA).
5. 21.1 mg/ml trastuzumab (Herceptin), IgG1K (Genentech and Biogen).

2.4 Buffers and Kits

1. MACS buffer: 0.5% HSA + 2 mM EDTA in PBS.
2. NK cell isolation kit (MACS Miltenyi Biotec, Germany).

2.5 Supplies

1. 96-well U bottom culture plates.
2. 96-well Luma plates (Perkin Elmer, USA).
3. Counting slide.
4. Falcon tubes 15 ml and 50 ml.
5. Pipet tips 0.5–1000 μl.
6. Reagent reservoirs.
7. Round-bottom polystyrene tubes 5 ml (BD Falcon, USA).

8. Serological pipettes 5 ml, 10 ml, 25 ml, and 50 ml.
9. SHIELDskin™ ORANGE NITRILE™ 260 gloves.
10. Tissue culture dish 35, 100 mm.
11. Tissue culture flask 25 and 75 cm^2.

2.6 Instruments

1. Centrifuge 5810.
2. Incubator BE200.
3. Light microscope DMLS.
4. Luna™ automated cell counter.
5. MACS magnet.
6. MACS column.
7. Multichannel pipette.
8. PipetBoy Pro.
9. Pipettes.
10. Scintillation counter 1450 Microbeta reader Trilux.
11. Vortexer Reax top.
12. Water bath GD100.

3 Methods

3.1 NK Cell Isolation

To use NK cells from fresh or previously frozen peripheral blood mononuclear cells (PBMCs), first you need to isolate and purify them. This can be done with the MACS NK cell isolation kit which includes a human NK cell biotin-antibody cocktail and a NK cell microbead cocktail. NK cells are isolated from PBMCs by immunomagnetic negative selection. Unwanted cells (monocytes, B cells, T cells) are labeled with antibody complexes, and magnetic particles and the target cells remain unlabeled. Magnetically labeled cells are then separated from NK cells with a magnet and by collecting the flow-through after pipetting the cells into a MACS column. The flow-through contains the NK cells since they do not bind to the column.

The protocol followed to perform the NK isolation is the one provided by MACS Miltenyi Biotec [12] (*see* **Note 1**).

1. Prepare MACS buffer and store it in the fridge at 4 °C (*see* **Note 2**).
2. For the magnetic labeling, prepare cells and determine cell number. For optimal isolation, it is important to obtain a single-cell suspension before the labeling by spinning down the cells at 400 × *g* for 5 min. After that, count the cells (*see* **Note 3**).

Table 1
MACS columns and magnets that can be used for NK cell isolation

Column	Max number of labeled cells	Max number of total cells	Magnet
MS	10^7	2×10^8	MiniMACS, OctoMACS
LS	10^8	2×10^9	MidiMACS, QuadroMACS
autoMACS	2×10^8	4×10^9	autoMACS Pro

3. Centrifuge again and resuspend cell pellet in 40 μl of MACS buffer per 10^7 total cells.
4. Add 10 μl of NK cell biotin-antibody cocktail per 10^7 total cells. Mix well by pipetting up and down, and incubate for 5 min in the fridge at 4 °C (*see* **Note 4**).
5. Next, add 30 μl of MACS buffer per 10^7 total cells and 20 μl of NK cell microbead cocktail per 10^7 total cells. Mix well and incubate for 10 min at 4 °C.
6. Proceed to subsequent magnetic cell separation. Place column in the magnetic field of a suitable MACS magnet. For details about which column can be used, *see* Table 1. A minimum of 500 μl is required for magnetic separation. If necessary, add MACS buffer to the cell suspension (*see* **Note 5**).
7. Prepare column by rinsing with the appropriate amount of buffer. For the MS column, use 500 μl and for the LS column, 3 ml. Always wait until the column reservoir is empty before proceeding to the next step.
8. Apply cell suspension onto the column. Collect the flow-through in a 15 ml falcon tube, containing the unlabeled cells. This fraction corresponds to the enriched NK cells.
9. When the column is empty, wash it with the appropriate amount of MACS buffer. For the MS column, use 500 μl and for the LS column, 3 ml. Collect unlabeled cells that pass through, and combine them with the effluent from the previous step (this fraction might contain some leftovers of NK cells).
10. If you want to collect the magnetically labeled cells (optionally), remove the column from the magnet, and place it on a suitable falcon tube. Pipette the appropriate amount of buffer onto the column: 1 ml for the MS column and 5 ml for the LS column. Immediately flush out the magnetically labeled non-NK cells by firmly pushing the plunger into the column.

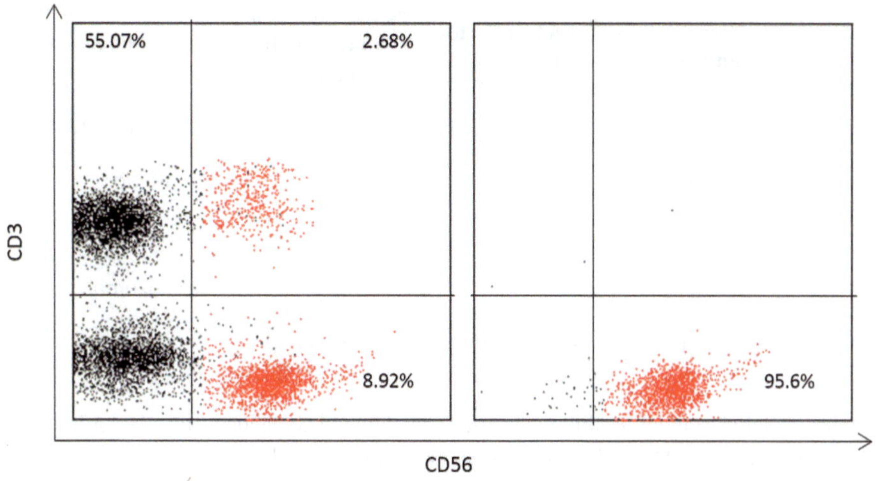

Fig. 3 Example of a purification using the NK cell isolation kit. Flow cytometry data from PBMCs (left) and isolated NK cells (right). Around 9% of the PBMCs are NK cells, which are characterized to be $CD56^+$ and $CD3^-$ as shown here

11. After the NK isolation, count the cells and centrifuge them at 400 × *g* for 5 min.
12. Resuspend NK cells in 5 ml IMDM +10% FCS, and transfer them to a T25 flask. Keep the cells in an incubator at 37 °C and 5% CO_2 (*see* **Note 6**).
13. If the cells are used the next day in a cytotoxicity assay, stimulate them with 1 μl IL-2 500 U/ml. First, prepare 1 μl of IL-2 18×10^5 U/ml in 4 ml phosphate buffered saline (PBS) to have the right concentration (*see* **Note 7**).
14. To check the purity of the isolated NK cells, the cells can be fluorescently stained with the CD3 and CD56 antibodies and analyzed by flow cytometry. An example of NK cell purification can be seen in Fig. 3.

3.2 Chromium Release Assay

1. For this experiment, NK cells are used as the effector cells. These cells can be isolated from fresh or frozen PBMCs as described above. The NK cells used are previously stimulated overnight with 500 U/ml of IL-2 (*see* **Note 7**).
2. Collect target cells. If needed, treat with versene solution for 10 min at 37 °C to detach the cells from the flask. Check whether the cells are detached with a microscope (*see* **Note 8**).
3. Wash the cells with PBS for 5 min at 400 × *g*. Resuspend the cells in 3 ml PBS, and count them with trypan blue/automated cell counter.
4. After counting the cells, prepare the amount of target cells that are needed (5×10^3 cells/well) in 3 ml of PBS. Because some cells might die during the labeling with radioactive chromium,

	Target + effector	Target + effector + IgG1 1 μg/ml	Target + effector + Trastuzumab 1 μg/ml	Max killing
	1 2 3	4 5 6	7 8 9	10 11 12
A	9:1	9:1	9:1	no ab
B	3:1	3:1	3:1	IgG1
C	1:1	1:1	1:1	trastuzumab
D	Target alone	Target alone	Target alone	

Fig. 4 Example of plate layout for a cytotoxicity assay with different conditions. The effector/target ratios used are the following: 9:1, 3:1, and 1:1. IgG1 is used as the isotype control

label two times more cells than needed to be sure to have enough cells. For each well you will need 5×10^3 cells. Therefore, for a whole 96-well plate, you will need 4.8×10^5 cells, and thus 10^6 cells should be labeled. For an example of a plate for a cytotoxicity assay, *see* Fig. 4. Transfer the cells to a round-bottom polystyrene tube.

5. Wash the cells again with PBS for 5 min at 400 × *g*, and resuspend them in 40 μl warm fetal calf serum (FCS) with 10 μl DNase at 400 U/ml (*see* **Note 9**).
6. Before starting to use the radioactive isotope, monitor background radioactivity levels. Take the precautions needed to work with radioactivity! (*see* **Note 10**).
7. Vortex the cells before adding ^{51}Cr. Add 10 μl of Cr^{51}/million cells to the tube with the cells. Monitor the levels of radioactivity after working with radioisotopes.
8. Incubate for 1 h in the incubator at 37 °C in the radioactivity room.
9. In the meantime, collect the stimulated NK cells, pellet them 5 min at 400 × *g*, and wash them with PBS. This step is done to remove the IL-2 of the cells.
10. Resuspend the effector cells in RPMI containing 10% FCS or another appropriate medium. Next, count the cells with trypan blue/automated cell counter.
11. Since you want to evaluate the cytotoxicity of NK cells, it is useful to use different ratios of effector cells. In this case, we decided to use the following E:T ratios: 9:1, 3:1, and 1:1 (Fig. 4). For example, for the highest ratio, you will need 9 times 5×10^3 cells per well. This amount can be further diluted to obtain the other ratios.

12. In each well, there should be 100 μl effector cells and 100 μl target cells. Thus, in the case of the ratio 9:1, the concentration of NK cells should be 4.5×10^5 cells/ml. This number of cells can be further diluted in RPMI +10% FCS medium to obtain the other concentrations. Prepare the right concentration of effector cells of the highest ratio in RPMI +10% FCS medium.
13. Add 100 μl RPMI medium to the rows of a 96-well U bottom plate where the serially dilutions will be made. As it can be seen from Fig. 3, it will be rows B–C (ratio 3:1, 1:1). Also add 100 μl medium to the wells where there will only be target cells (target alone). The target alone wells are used as a control for spontaneous killing. Make triplicates of each condition (*see* **Note 11**).
14. Plate 200 μl NK cells with the concentration of the highest ratio (in this case, 4.5×10^5 cells/ml for a 9:1 ratio). Serially dilute the effector cells in row A (ratio 9:1) to obtain densities of 1.5×10^5 cells/ml (ratio 3:1) and 0.5×10^5 cells/ml (ratio 1:1). This can be done by transferring 100 μl of NK cells ratio 9:1 to the 6:1 ratio wells and resuspending well. With the same tips, transfer 100 μl of NK cells ratio 3:1 to the 1:1 ratio wells. Resuspend and throw away 100 μl from the wells with the lowest ratio (ratio 1:1).
15. To calculate the killing of target cells, it is necessary to compare it with the maximum killing (control). Therefore, a detergent such as Triton X-100 or SDS can be used. Add 100 μl of 5% Triton X-100 in RPMI to the max. killing wells (Fig. 4) (*see* **Note 12**).
16. After the incubation of the target cells with ^{51}Cr, add 2 ml RPMI +10% FCS medium to the labeled cells, and centrifuge for 4 min at $500 \times g$.
17. For all the subsequent steps, discard waste in a special radioactive-labeled container. Discard the supernatant (radioactive waste), vortex the cells, and resuspend them in 3 ml medium. Wash again and resuspend cells in 2 ml RPMI.
18. Count target cells with trypan blue/automated cell counter, and resuspend them in RPMI + 10% FCS medium at a concentration of 0.5×10^5 cells/ml (5×10^3 cells/well, 100 μl/well).
19. Depending on the different conditions that you want to test, divide the cells in different tubes (for each condition). In the example of Fig. 4, there are three different conditions: effector cells + target cells, effector cells + target cells and isotype control, and effector cells + target cells and trastuzumab (*see* **Note 13**).
20. Add trastuzumab (from 21.1 mg/ml stock solution) to a final concentration of 10 μg/ml, or add the isotype control IgG1

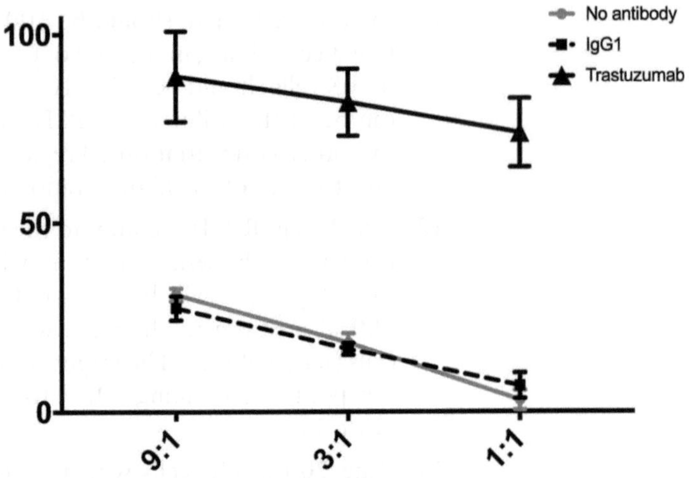

Fig. 5 Example of cytotoxicity assay with NK cells in combination with trastuzumab. The percentage of killing shown here is after overnight incubation

(from 5.3 mg/ml stock solution) to a final concentration of 10 μg/ml to the tubes/6-well plate (*see* **Notes 14** and **15**).

21. Add 100 μl target cells to each well and incubate for 4/18 h in 5% CO_2 at 37 °C (*see* **Note 16**).
22. Remove 20 μl supernatant with a multichannel after 4 h and 25 μl after 18 h, transfer to a 96-well Luma plate, and let it dry overnight. Resuspend *only* the cells of the max killing before transferring them to the Luma plate to be sure to have the highest killing (*see* **Note 17**).
23. Read plates in the microbeta plate reader with the non-phenol red protocol (*see* **Note 18**).
24. The percentage of killing can be calculated with the following formula by averaging counts from triplicate wells:

$$\text{Lysis}\,(\%) = \frac{\text{Experimental Cr}^{51}\text{ release} - \text{Spontaneous Cr}^{51}\text{ release}}{\text{Maximum Cr}^{51}\text{ release} - \text{Spontaneous Cr}^{51}\text{ release}} \times 100$$

25. Plot the percentage of killing at each E:T ratio, and compare it with the controls. Effective ADCC can be observed when killing is significantly increased in the presence of trastuzumab as compared to the controls (Fig. 5).

4 Notes

1. Most of the times, the labeled fraction of cells represents the majority of the total cells, as it is the case with NK cells which represent 5–10% of the PBMCs. So, to avoid blocking the column, do not exceed the max number of labeled cells per column which is indicated in Table 1. Therefore, it is important to estimate the number of labeled cells in the sample, to split the sample if necessary and to use the appropriate separation column.
2. Depending on the number of cells you want to isolate, you will need a different amount of MACS buffer. It is practical to make more MACS buffer than what you need so you can use it for other NK cell isolations. MACS buffer can be stored at 4 °C for up to 1 month.
3. The volumes shown in the protocol are for up to 10^7 total cells. When you have less cells, use the same volumes as indicated. When working with higher cell numbers, scale up all reagent and total volumes accordingly.
4. Store the biotin-antibody cocktail and the microbead cocktail at 2–8 °C protected from light. Work fast, and keep cells and solutions cold as much as possible (2–8 °C). During the incubation times, incubate always in the fridge at 4 °C. Keep the MACS column cold until it is needed.
5. If you are not sure which column you should use, then the best one to use to avoid blocking of the column is the LS column. It can be used even though the number of total cells is less than 2×10^8. This will lead to a better separation of the cells.
6. Leave the cells in a vertical position in the incubator to increase growing and viability of NK cells.
7. A low concentration of IL-2 is added to keep the cells activated but not too much since we want to mimic physiological conditions, and we do not want to overstimulate the cells.
8. This step is only needed if you have adherent cells. Trypsin or a combination of trypsin with versene can also be used to trypsinize the cells. To split the cells that are in culture, we use trypsin, but prior to and ADCC experiment, we prefer to use versene since it is milder, and it does not damage the extracellular receptors.
9. DNase is used to prevent aggregation of the cells. If the stock solution is more concentrated, it should be diluted first with PBS. The recommended solvent for DNase is filtered Milli-Q water. Solutions can be kept for 2 days at 2 to 8 °C and for 1 month at −15 to −20 °C. For best results, prepare appropriate aliquots, and avoid repeated freezing and thawing [13].

10. Using suitable gloves and working behind a protective shield will reduce the risk of internal contamination. Since the activity is proportional to the inverse of the square of the distance, keeping distance from the source will reduce the activity of chromium considerably. Other precautions that can be taken are shortening the exposure time and using adequate shielding. Since chromium is a γ-emitter, lead would be a proper shielding. From now on, materials that are contaminated with ^{51}Cr should be discarded in a special bin clearly labeled and handled according to local regulations.
11. To avoid having variation between the samples, it is recommended to use a multichannel pipette.
12. Triton X-100 20% was already prepared and stored in the fridge for other cytotoxicity assays. This solution was made by diluting Triton X-100 in RPMI medium. Because of its high viscosity, it can be quite difficult to dissolve it. Therefore, putting the solution in a water bath at 37 °C during a few minutes can help solving this problem.
13. To divide the target cells so the different antibodies can be added, you can use a 6-well plate instead of using different tubes. The antibody that is then pipetted can be well mixed in the solution. It is also more practical since you can pipette the cells directly from the 6-well plate to the 96-well plate with a multichannel pipette.
14. The amount of antibody needed depends on the concentration of target cells that will be used.
15. If another antibody is used to induce ADCC, then the correspondent IgG isotype control should be used.
16. To prevent evaporation of the wells, you can add PBS to the surrounding wells.
17. Part of the supernatant of the cytotoxicity assay can be stored at −20 °C and used for an ELISA.
18. Let the machine warm up for 600 min before starting to measure.

References

1. Yamashita M, Kitano S, Aikawa H, Kuchiba A, Hayashi M, Yamamoto N et al (2016) A novel method for evaluating antibody-dependent cell-mediated cytotoxicity by flowcytometry using cryopreserved human peripheral blood mononuclear cells. Sci Rep 6:19772. https://doi.org/10.1038/srep19772
2. Morvan MG, Lanier LL (2016) NK cells and cancer: you can teach innate cells new tricks. Nat Rev Cancer 16(1):7–19. https://doi.org/10.1038/nrc.2015.5
3. Abbas A, Lichtman AH, Pillai S (2014) Cellular and molecular immunology, 8th edn. Elsevier
4. Altfeld M, Fadda L, Frleta D, Bhardwaj N (2011) DCs and NK cells: critical effectors in the immune response to HIV-1. Nat Rev Immunol 11:176–186

5. Slamon DJ, Leyland-Jones B, Shak S, Fuchs H, Paton V, Bajamonde A et al (2001) Use of chemotherapy plus a monoclonal antibody against HER2 for metastatic breast cancer that overexpresses HER2. N Engl J Med 344 (11):783–792. https://doi.org/10.1056/nejm200103153441101
6. Yu L, Wang Y, Yao Y, Li W, Lai Q, Li J et al (2014) Eradication of growth of HER2-positive ovarian cancer with trastuzumab-DM1, an antibody-cytotoxic drug conjugate in mouse xenograft model. Int J Gynecol Cancer 24(7):1158–1164. https://doi.org/10.1097/igc.0000000000000179
7. Tak W, Mak MES (2006) MHC: the major histocompatibility complex. The immune response. Elsevier
8. Brunner KT, Mauel J, Cerottini JC, Chapuis B (1968) Quantitative assay of the lytic action of immune lymphoid cells on 51-Cr-labelled allogeneic target cells in vitro; inhibition by isoantibody and by drugs. Immunology 14 (2):181–196
9. Kiessling R, Klein E (1973) Cytotoxic potential of mouse spleen cells on H-2 antibody-treated target cells. J Exp Med 137 (2):527–532
10. Zaritskaya L, Shurin MR, Sayers TJ, Malyguine AM (2010) New flow cytometric assays for monitoring cell-mediated cytotoxicity. Expert Rev Vaccines 9(6):601–616. https://doi.org/10.1586/erv.10.49
11. Adams S, Alving B, Anderson KC, AuBuchon JP, Bandarenko N, Barrett J et al (2007) Contributors. In: Blood banking and transfusion medicine, 2nd edn. Churchill Livingstone, Philadelphia, pp vii–xiii. https://doi.org/10.1016/B978-0-443-06981-9.50003-X
12. NK cell isolation kit. Miltenyi Biotec. http://www.miltenyibiotec.com/en/products-and-services/macs-cell-separation/cell-separation-reagents/microbeads-and-isolation-kits/nk-cells/nk-cell-isolation-kit-human.aspx
13. DNase I Recombinant. Sigma-Aldrich https://www.sigmaaldrich.com/catalog/product/roche/04716728001?lang=en&region=GB&gclid=EAIaIQobChMIktKWzPmq2AIVAhwbCh1bVQpHEAAYASAAEgLO1fD_BwE

Chapter 13

Evaluating Antibody-Dependent Cell-Mediated Cytotoxicity by Flow Cytometry

Irene van der Haar Àvila, Patricia Marmol, Jeannette Cany, Rolf Kiessling, and Yago Pico de Coaña

Abstract

Antibody-dependent cell-mediated cytotoxicity (ADCC) is a mechanism in which immune cell activation is induced by the cross-linking of CD16 with the Fc region of antibodies that at the same time bind specifically to cell surface antigens. ADCC stimulates the secretion of perforin, granzymes, and cytokines leading to lysis of the malignant cells. Natural killer (NK) cells express the CD16 receptor and can therefore be activated by ADCC to kill tumor cells. To study the cytotoxicity of NK cells against cancer cells, an ADCC-based assay is described: the flow cytometry-based cytotoxicity assay. In this method, the antibody trastuzumab, which binds specifically to HER2-positive malignant cells, is used to trigger ADCC.

Key words Antibody cell-mediated cytotoxicity, Natural killer cells, Trastuzumab, Flow cytometry

1 Introduction

Recently, there has been rapid progress in the field of clinical immunotherapy. In particular, the use of monoclonal antibodies (mAbs) for cancer therapy is one of the most effective strategies for treating cancer patients. Such mAbs can kill tumor cells by (1) blocking the function of the target molecule, (2) mediating the delivery of cytotoxic drugs, (3) affecting the tumor vasculature or stroma, and/or (4) triggering immune-mediated cell-killing mechanisms, such as antibody-dependent cell-mediated cytotoxicity (ADCC) [1]. ADCC occurs when the Fc-γ (CD16) receptor of effector immune cells becomes activated after interaction with antibodies. Natural killer (NK) cells, macrophages, and granulocytes express the CD16 receptor that recognizes the Fc region of IgG antibodies [2]. These antibodies can bind specifically to antigens that are expressed on malignant cells. At the same time they can cross-link with the Fc receptors, triggering cell activation and

Yago Pico de Coaña (ed.), *Immune Checkpoint Blockade: Methods and Protocols*, Methods in Molecular Biology, vol. 1913, https://doi.org/10.1007/978-1-4939-8979-9_13, © Springer Science+Business Media, LLC, part of Springer Nature 2019

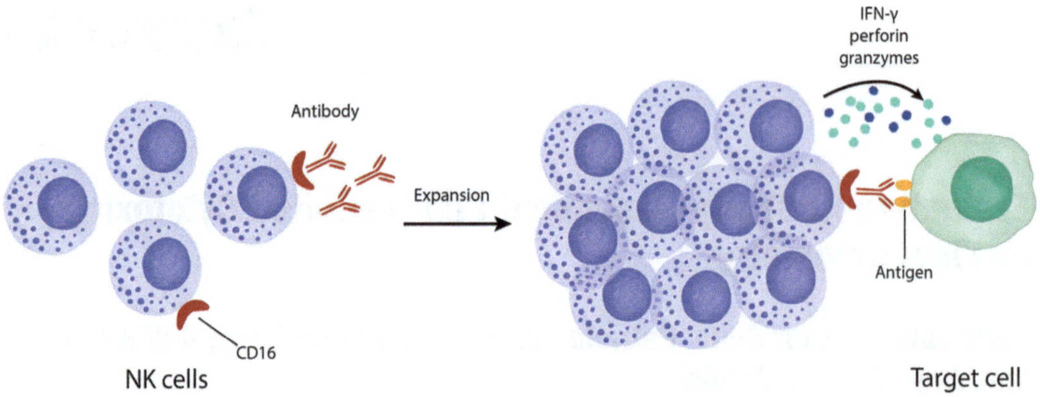

Fig. 1 Schematic representation of antibody-dependent cellular cytotoxicity (ADCC) mediated by NK cells. Using a specific antibody that binds to the CD16 Fc receptors and to tumor-associated antigens, NK cells become activated via antibody-dependent cell-mediated cytotoxicity inducing IFNγ, perforin, and granzymes release (Adapted from Morvan et al. [2])

secretion of cytokines such as IFNγ and granzymes, resulting in target cell lysis (Fig. 1) [3, 4].

There are already some clinically approved antibodies where ADCC has shown to participate as the active mechanism. One example is trastuzumab (Herceptin), a humanized mAb directed against the extracellular domain of the HER2 receptor [1]. Trastuzumab is widely used in the treatment of HER2-positive cancers, including breast cancer and ovarian cancer, among others [5, 6]. It binds to the CD16 receptor and to the HER2/neu receptor of malignant cells inducing immune-mediated responses.

The cytotoxicity of NK cells mediated by antibody immunotherapy can be studied by flow cytometry or by chromium (^{51}Cr) release assays. With flow cytometry, living and dead target and effector cells can be detected and quantified based on differential staining by fluorescent dyes [1]. CFSE (carboxyfluorescein succinimidyl ester) can be used as a dye to specifically label the target cell population to distinguish target and effector cells.

In ^{51}Cr release assays, the release of radioactive chromium from pre-labeled target cells is measured. The cells take up the radioisotope which then binds intracellularly to macromolecules. As long as the labeled cells are viable, the ^{51}Cr-macromolecule complexes remain contained in the cell because they cannot cross the membrane [7]. When the cells are lysed, the contents of the cell are released and therefore also the radioactive chromium, which can then be measured. This method has long been the most widely used technique for measuring cell-mediated cytotoxicity [1, 8] and was the first method used to evaluate ADCC [9]. The advantages of using chromium release assays are that less cells are needed and thus more conditions can be tested. However, it has some disadvantages, such as toxicity for target cells, low sensitivity, labeling irregularities, and the generation of radioactive waste [10]. In contrast, flow cytometry-based cytotoxicity assays are more sensitive and reproducible, and both live and dead populations of target and effector cells can be visualized. It is also possible to perform immunophenotyping at the single-cell level. Since these cells are not cultured with toxic isotopes, long-term cultures can be maintained, and thus long-term effects on cytotoxicity can be studied [1]. However, for the flow cytometry assays, a higher number of cells are needed.

Here, we describe a flow cytometry-based assay to evaluate ADCC in NK cells with the antibody trastuzumab.

2 Materials

2.1 Cells

1. Fresh/frozen PBMCs.
2. Purified NK cells (or other effector cells).
3. Target cells (SkBr3 or other cell lines).

2.2 Reagents and Chemicals

1. 7AAD live/dead cell marker (Sigma, St Louis, USA).
2. CellTrace™ CFSE Cell Proliferation Kit (Thermo Fisher scientific, Göteborg, Sweden).
3. DC medium CellGro GMP + 2% HSA (human serum albumin).
4. 99.5% ethanol.
5. FCS (fetal calf serum).
6. IMDM (Iscove's modified Dulbecco's medium) + 10% FCS (fetal calf serum).
7. PBS (phosphate-buffered saline).
8. RPMI 1640 (Roswell Park Memorial Institute) + 10% FCS (fetal calf serum) + Penicillin/Streptomycin.
9. Trypan blue.
10. 0.05% trypsin-EDTA.

2.3 Antibodies and Cytokines

1. CD3-PO-conjugated antibody (Invitrogen, UK).
2. CD56-PE-Cy7-conjugated antibody (BioLegend, San Diego, USA).
3. 18×10^5 U/ml IL-2 (Novartis, Copenhagen, Denmark).
4. 5.3 mg/ml isotype control, hIgG1 (BMS, NY, USA).
5. 21.1 mg/ml trastuzumab (Herceptin), IgG1K (Genentech and Biogen).

2.4 Buffers and Kits

1. FACS buffer: 1% HSA in PBS.
2. MACS buffer: 0.5% HSA + 2 mM EDTA in PBS.
3. NK cell isolation kit (MACS Miltenyi Biotec, Germany).

2.5 Supplies

1. 96-well flat bottom culture plates.
2. Counting slide.
3. Falcon tubes 15 ml and 50 ml.
4. Micronics tubes.
5. Pipet tips 0.5–1000 μl.
6. Reagent reservoirs.
7. Serological pipettes 5 ml, 10 ml, 25 ml, and 50 ml.
8. Tissue culture flasks 25 and 75 cm^2.

2.6 Instruments

1. Centrifuge 5810.
2. FACS LSRII flow cytometer.
3. Incubator BE200.
4. Light microscope DMLS.
5. Luna™ automated cell counter.
6. MACS magnet.
7. MACS column.
8. Multichannel pipette.
9. PipetBoy Pro.
10. Pipettes.
11. Vortexer Reax top.
12. Water bath GD100.

3 Methods

3.1 NK Cell Isolation

To use NK cells from fresh or previously frozen peripheral blood mononuclear cells (PBMCs), first you need to isolate and purify them. This can be done with the MACS NK cell isolation kit which includes a human NK cell Biotin-Antibody Cocktail and a NK cell MicroBead Cocktail. NK cells are isolated from PBMCs by immunomagnetic negative selection. Unwanted cells (monocytes, B cells, T cells) are labeled with antibody complexes, and magnetic particles and the target cells remain unlabeled. Magnetically labeled cells are then separated from NK cells with a magnet and by collecting the flow-through after pipetting the cells into a MACS column. The flow-through contains the NK cells since they do not bind to the column.

The protocol followed to perform the NK isolation is the one provided by MACS Miltenyi Biotec [11] (*see* **Note 1**).

1. Prepare MACS buffer and store it in the fridge at 4 °C (*see* **Note 2**).
2. For the magnetic labeling, prepare cells and determine cell number. For optimal isolation, it is important to obtain a single-cell suspension before the labeling by spinning down the cells at 400 × *g* for 5 min. After that, count the cells (*see* **Note 3**).
3. Centrifuge again and resuspend cell pellet in 40 μl of MACS buffer per 10^7 total cells.
4. Add 10 μl of NK Cell Biotin-Antibody Cocktail per 10^7 total cells. Mix well by pipetting up and down and incubate for 5 min in the fridge at 4 °C (*see* **Note 4**).
5. Next, add 30 μl of MACS buffer per 10^7 total cells and 20 μl of NK cell MicroBead Cocktail per 10^7 total cells. Mix well and incubate for 10 min at 4 °C.
6. Proceed to subsequent magnetic cell separation. Place column in the magnetic field of a suitable MACS magnet. For details about which column can be used, see Table 1. A minimum of 500 μl is required for magnetic separation. If necessary, add MACS buffer to the cell suspension (*see* **Note 5**).
7. Prepare column by rinsing with the appropriate amount of buffer. For the MS column, use 500 μl and for the LS column, 3 ml. Always wait until the column reservoir is empty before proceeding to the next step.
8. Apply cell suspension onto the column. Collect the flow-through in a 15 ml falcon tube, containing the unlabeled cells. This fraction corresponds to the enriched NK cells.
9. When the column is empty, wash it with the appropriate amount of MACS buffer. For the MS column, use 500 μl and for the LS column, 3 ml. Collect unlabeled cells that pass through, and combine them with the effluent from the previous step (this fraction might contain some leftovers of NK cells).

Table 1
MACS columns and magnets that can be used for NK cell isolation

Column	Max. number of labeled cells	Max. number of total cells	Magnet
MS	10^7	2×10^8	MiniMACS, OctoMACS
LS	10^8	2×10^9	MidiMACS, QuadroMACS
autoMACS	2×10^8	4×10^9	autoMACS Pro

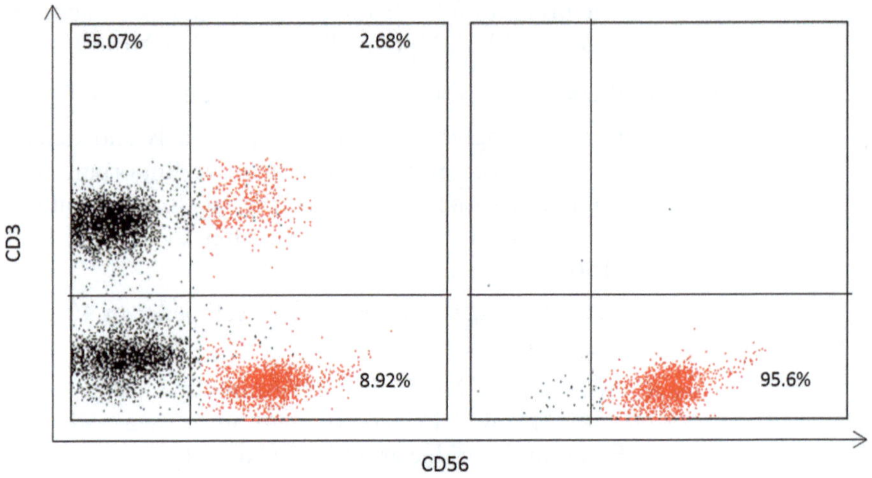

Fig. 2 Example of a purification using the NK cell isolation kit. Flow cytometry data from PBMCs (left) and isolated NK cells (right). Around 9% of the PBMCs are NK cells, which are characterized to be CD56$^+$ and CD3$^-$ as it is shown here

10. If you want to collect the magnetically labeled cells (optionally), remove the column from the magnet and place it on a suitable falcon tube. Pipette the appropriate amount of buffer onto the column: 1 ml for the MS column and 5 ml for the LS column. Immediately flush out the magnetically labeled non-NK cells by firmly pushing the plunger into the column.
11. After the NK isolation, count the cells and centrifuge them at 400 × *g* for 5 min.
12. Resuspend NK cells in 5 ml IMDM +10% FCS and transfer them to a T25 flask. Keep the cells in an incubator at 37 °C and 5% CO_2 (*see* **Note 6**).
13. If the cells are used the next day in a cytotoxicity assay, stimulate them with 1 μl IL-2500 U/ml. First, prepare 1 μl of IL-2 18×10^5 U/ml in 4 ml phosphate-buffered saline (PBS) to have the right concentration (*see* **Note 7**).
14. To check the purity of the isolated NK cells, the cells can be fluorescently stained with the CD3 and CD56 antibodies and analyzed by flow cytometry. An example of NK cell purification can be seen in Fig. 2.

3.2 Flow Cytometry-Based Cytotoxicity

1. For this experiment, NK cells are used as the effector cells. These cells can be isolated from fresh or frozen PBMCs as described above. The NK cells used are previously stimulated overnight with 500 U/ml of IL-2 (*see* **Note 7**).
2. Collect target cells in a 15 ml falcon tube. If it is needed, treat with versene solution for 10 min at 37 °C to detach the cells from the flask. Check whether the cells are detached with a microscope (*see* **Note 8**).

	Target + effector			Target + effector + IgG1 1 μg/ml			Target + effector + Trastuzumab 1 μg/ml			Max killing		
	1	2	3	4	5	6	7	8	9	10	11	12
A		9:1			9:1			9:1			no ab	
B		3:1			3:1			3:1			IgG1	
C		1:1			1:1			1:1			trastuzumab	
D		Target alone			Target alone			Target alone				

Fig. 3 Example of plate layout for a cytotoxicity assay with different conditions. The effector/target ratios used are the following: 9:1, 3:1, and 1:1. Rituximab is used as a control for ADCC

3. Wash the cells with PBS for 5 min at 400 × *g* and resuspend the cells in 5 ml PBS.
4. In order to visualize and distinguish the target cells from the effector cells with flow cytometry, you need to label fluorescently either the target or the effector cells. This can be done with the CFSE Cell Proliferation Kit. Prepare a 1:500 dilution of CFSE: 2 μl CFSE 5 mM in 1 ml PBS (end concentration is 10 μM) (*see* **Note 9**).
5. Centrifuge the cells for 5 min at 400 × *g* and resuspend cell pellet in 270 μl PBS.
6. Add 30 μl of 10 μM CFSE to the cells, mix gently with a pipette and incubate 10 min at 37 °C.
7. After the incubation, add 300 μl of FCS and agitate 1 min in a water bath at 37 °C.
8. Wash the cells with 10 ml PBS for 5 min at 400 × *g* and resuspend pellet in 5 ml PBS. Count the cells with trypan blue/automated cell counter (*see* **Note 10**).
9. After counting the cells, determine the amount of target cells that are needed (2–3 × 10^4 cells/well). To analyze the results of the cytotoxicity assay by flow cytometry, you need more cells than by chromium release. In this case, for each well you will need 3 × 10^4 cells. Therefore, for a whole 96-well plate, you will need approx. 3 × 10^6 cells. When the target cells are plated the day before, using 2 × 10^4 cells per well is enough because they will grow overnight. For an example of a plate for a cytotoxicity assay, see Fig. 3.
10. In every well you will plate 100 μl target cells, so prepare the cells at a concentration of 3 × 10^5 cells/ml in appropriate medium such as RPMI +10% FCS or IMDM +10% FCS in a 15 ml falcon tube (*see* **Notes 11** and **12**).

11. Plate 100 μl of target cell in a 96-well flat bottom plate. Do not forget to plate target cells without effector cells as a control (target alone). Make triplicates of each condition (*see* **Notes 13** and **14**).
12. In the case of using adherent cells, incubate them overnight at 37 °C and 5% CO_2. Otherwise, start preparing the effector cells (*see* **Notes 15** and **16**).
13. To prepare the effector cells, collect the stimulated NK cells in 15 ml falcon tube, pellet them 5 min at 400 g and wash them with PBS. This step is done to remove the IL-2 of the cells.
14. Resuspend the effector cells in appropriate medium. Next, count the cells with trypan blue/automated cell counter (*see* **Note 17**).
15. To study the cytotoxicity of NK cells, it is better to use different ratios of effector cells. In this case, we decided to use the following E:T ratios: 9:1, 3:1, and 1:1 (Fig. 3). For example, for the highest ratio, you will need 9 times 3×10^4 cells per well (*see* **Notes 18** and **19**).
16. In each well, there should be 100 μl effector cells and 100 μl target cells. Thus, in the case of the ratio 9:1, the concentration of NK cells should be 2.7×10^6 cells/ml. This concentration is then further diluted with medium to obtain the other concentrations. Prepare the right concentration of effector cells of the highest ratio in DC medium + 2% HSA or another medium.
17. Make two successive dilutions 1:3 of the highest ratio NK cell suspension to obtain densities of 0.9×10^6 cells/ml (ratio 3:1) and 0.3×10^6 cells/ml (ratio 1:1) (*see* **Note 20**).
18. Add 10 μl trastuzumab or add 10 μl of the isotype control IgG1 to the correspondent wells. Use both antibodies at a concentration of 10 μg/ml. Add 10 μl PBS to the wells where there is no antibody added to have the same volume everywhere (*see* **Notes 21–24**).
19. (Optional) In the case of adherent cells, incubate the cells 30 min at 37 °C. Carefully remove 100 μl of supernatant and gently wash the cells with PBS. Put back 100 μl medium to the cells (*see* **Note 25**).
20. Plate 100 μl NK cells per well (i.e., 2.7×10^5, 0.9×10^5, and 0.3×10^5 NKs per well). Add 100 μl medium to control wells (target alone) to have 200 μl as a final volume in all wells (*see* **Note 26**).
21. Incubate the cells overnight at 37 °C and 5% CO_2 (*see* **Notes 16** and **27**).

22. After overnight incubation, the killing is analyzed. Prepare Micronics tubes for cytotoxicity assay acquisition with flow cytometry (one tube for each well) (*see* **Notes 28** and **29**).
23. For nonadherent target cells, resuspend each well with a multichannel pipette, and transfer all the cell suspension into the Micronics tubes. In each Micronics tube, add 75 μl FACS buffer containing 7AAD (diluted 1:500) (*see* **Note 30**).
24. For adherent target cells, resuspend gently and transfer the cell suspension into the Micronics tubes. Add 70 μl PBS in each well, resuspend and transfer back in Micronics tubes. Add 30 μl trypsin or versene in each well, and incubate 5 min at 37 °C. Check that cells are well detached using the microscope. Add 50 μl PBS to the wells, pipet up and down gently, and transfer 80 μl into the tubes.
25. Trypsinize again for 5 min at 37 °C. Add 60 μl back from Micronics tubes to the wells and pipette up and down to detach and resuspend the cells. Retransfer 90 μl of the cell suspension to the Micronics tubes.
26. In each tube, add 10 μl FACS buffer containing 7AAD (diluted 1:25).
27. Vortex gently all the tubes and acquire data on flow cytometer. Run each sample for 1 min. An overview of the gating strategy is shown in Fig. 4.
28. Target cell survival was calculated as follows (counts from triplicate wells are averaged):

$$\text{Viable target cells }(\%) = \frac{\text{Viable CFSE}^{+}\text{ target cells cocultured with NK cells}}{\text{Viable CFSE}^{+}\text{ targetalone cells}} \times 100$$

The percentage specific lysis was calculated as follows:

$$\text{Specific lysis }(\%) = 100 - \text{Viable target cells }(\%)$$

29. Plot the percentage of killing at each E:T ratio and compare with the controls. Effective ADCC can be observed when killing is significantly increased in the presence of trastuzumab as compared to the controls (Fig. 5).

4 Notes

1. Most of the times, the labeled fraction of cells represents the majority of the total cells, as it is the case with NK cells which represent 5–10% of the PBMCs. So, to avoid blocking the column, do not exceed the max. number of labeled cells per column which is indicated in Table 1. Therefore, it is important

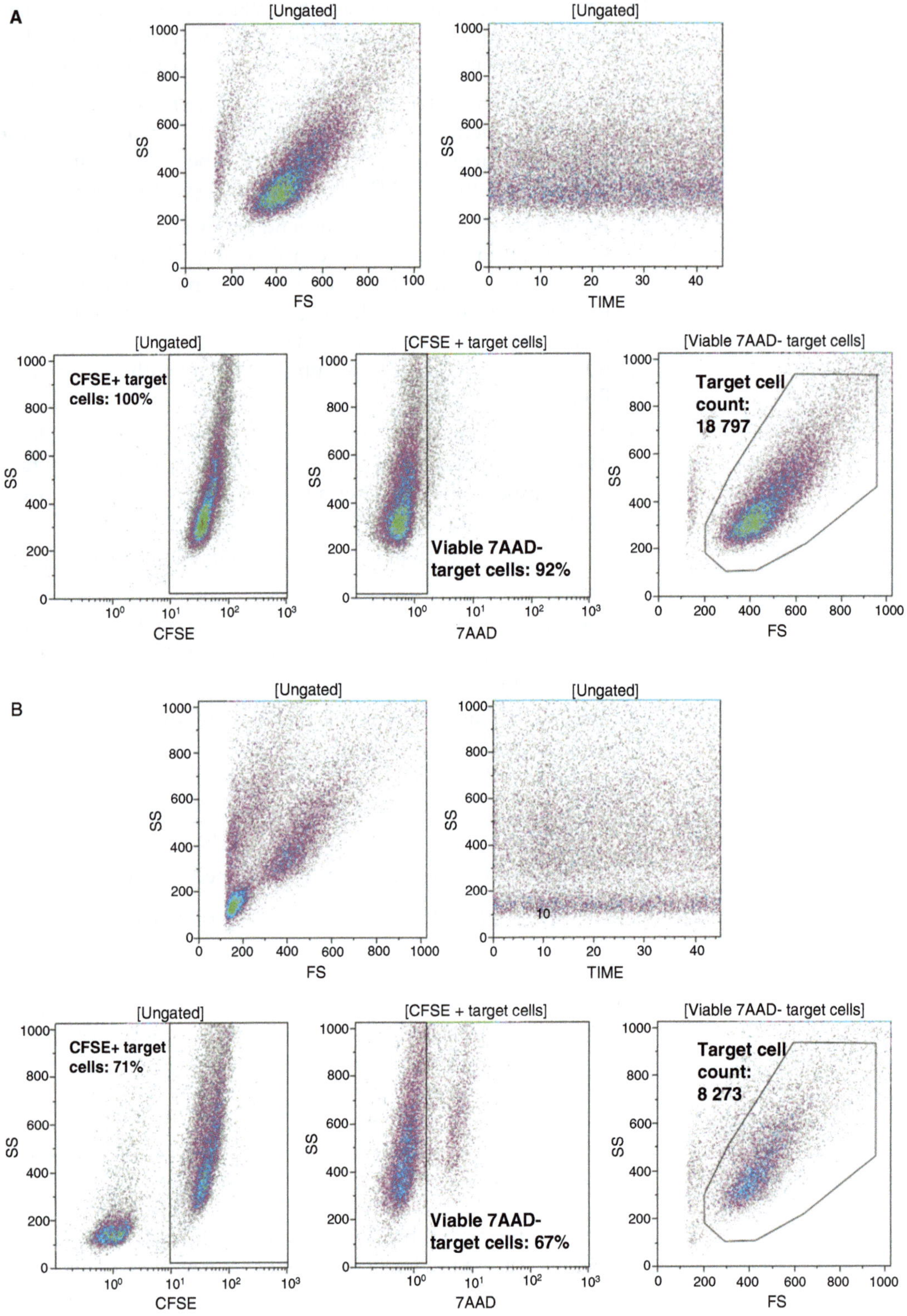

Fig. 4 Gating strategy of viable target cells. (**A**) Gating of CFSE$^+$ target cells alone. (**B**) Gating of CFSE$^+$ target cells with effector cells. Viable cells are 7AAD negative

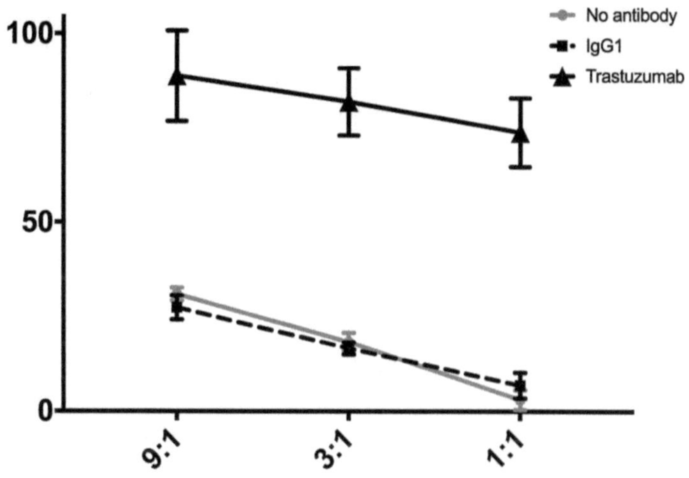

Fig. 5 Example of cytotoxicity assay with NK cells in combination with trastuzumab. The percentage of killing shown here is after overnight incubation

to estimate the number of labeled cells in the sample, to split the sample if necessary and to use the appropriate separation column.

2. Depending on the number of cells you want to isolate, you will need a different amount of MACS buffer. It is practical to make more MACS buffer than what you need so you can use it for other NK cell isolations. MACS buffer can be stored at 4 °C for up to 1 month.
3. The volumes shown in the protocol are for up to 10^7 total cells. When you have less cells, use the same volumes as indicated. When working with higher cell numbers, scale up all reagent and total volumes accordingly.
4. Store the Biotin-Antibody Cocktail and the MicroBead Cocktail at 2–8 °C protected from light. Work fast, and keep cells and solutions cold as much as possible (2–8 °C). During the incubation times, incubate always in the fridge at 4 °C. Keep the MACS column cold until it is needed.
5. If you are not sure which column you should use, then the best one to use to avoid blocking of the column is the LS column. It can be used even though the number of total cells is less than 2×10^8. This will lead to a better separation of the cells.
6. Leave the cells in a vertical position in the incubator to increase growing and viability of NK cells.
7. A low concentration of IL-2 is added to keep the cells activated, but not too much since we want to mimic physiological conditions and we do not want to overstimulate the cells.

8. This step is only needed if you have adherent cells. Trypsin or a combination of trypsin with versene can also be used to trypsinize the cells. To split the cells that are in culture, we use trypsin, but prior to an ADCC experiment, we prefer to use versene since it is milder and it does not damage the extracellular receptors.
9. CFSE is a fluorescent dye used in vitro and in vivo labeling of cells to visualize them by flow cytometry. It is non-toxic to cells and has long-term signal stability. Store CFSE in the freezer (−5 to −30 °C) and protect from light [12].
10. Cells can also be counted with flow cytometry which is more precise when having a high number of cells, but then the cells need to be incubated with the antibodies, and this takes more time.
11. Always prepare more cells than what you really need to have enough volume to pipet the cells into the plate. It is recommended to use a multichannel pipette to reduce variation between the samples. If you want to use a multichannel pipette, you have to keep in mind that you will have to transfer the cells to a reagent reservoir to be able to pipette. Therefore, you will need to have a greater volume.
12. The medium used to prepare target cells is the one used to culture these cells. Depending on the type of target cells, use IMDM medium or RPMI medium. Be consistent and use the same medium for the whole experiment.
13. To avoid having variation between the samples, it is recommended to use a multichannel pipette.
14. As a control for the killing with NK cells, other target cells that lack the protein targeted by the antibody can be used. In this case K562 cells are an ideal control because they are sensitive to NK killing, but do not express HER2.
15. Preparation of effector cells can be done together with the preparation of the target cells or during incubation/centrifugation steps.
16. To prevent evaporation of the wells, you can add PBS to the surrounding wells.
17. NK cells can be cultured in DC medium +2% HSA and thus for this experiment we used this medium. However, other media can be used such as RPMI or IMDM. Here again, you should be consistent and use the same medium for NK cells during the whole experiment.
18. The viability and the cytotoxicity of NK cells may vary from donor to donor.

19. Other E:T ratios can be chosen depending on the target cells that are used.
20. These dilutions can be made in falcon tubes with DC medium or other medium used for NK cells. Prepare more volume of each dilution to be able to transfer it to a reagent reservoir and thus to pipette it with a multichannel pipette.
21. If another antibody is used to induce ADCC, then the correspondent IgG isotype control should be used.
22. The amount of antibody needed depends on the number of wells. For example, if you have 40 wells and the end concentration should be 10 μg/ml in a 200 μl well, then there should be 2 μg Ab/well. This means that for 40 wells, you will need 80 μg of the antibody. Using the stock concentration of the antibody, you can calculate the volume needed of the antibody. This volume should then be filled up to 400 μl (for 40 wells) with PBS.
23. The antibody solutions can be prepared before starting the experiment and stored in the fridge or between incubation times. This saves time during the experiment.
24. As an extra control, you can add some wells without antibody as it is done in the chromium release assay.
25. This step is done because we saw that we had better results when the excess of antibody in adherent cells was removed. However, it is not a necessary step, and it should not be done with non-adherent cells because then you would remove also the target cells.
26. No max. killing is needed for this assay since the percentage of killing is calculated with the number of viable cells.
27. In this case only the overnight incubation is done because all the cells are needed for the flow cytometry. Otherwise there would not be enough events to measure. An extra plate with a 4 h incubation can be performed but then an even higher number of cells would be needed.
28. It is practical to put the Micronics tubes in a rack at the same place as where the samples are found in the 96-well plate. This makes it easier to transfer the cells from the plate to the Micronics tubes and it avoids confusions.
29. Part of the supernatant of the cytotoxicity assay can be stored at −20 °C and used for an ELISA.
30. Prepare the dilution of 7AAD before and keep it on ice. 7AAD is used as a live/dead cell marker for flow cytometry. It is needed to determine the number of viable cells after the cytotoxicity assay.

References

1. Yamashita M, Kitano S, Aikawa H, Kuchiba A, Hayashi M, Yamamoto N, Tamura K, Hamada A (2016) A novel method for evaluating antibody-dependent cell-mediated cytotoxicity by flowcytometry using cryopreserved human peripheral blood mononuclear cells. Sci Rep 6:19772. https://doi.org/10.1038/srep19772
2. Morvan MG, Lanier LL (2016) NK cells and cancer: you can teach innate cells new tricks. Nat Rev Cancer 16(1):7–19. https://doi.org/10.1038/nrc.2015.5
3. Abbas A, Lichtman AH, Pillai S (2014) Cellular and molecular immunology. 8th edn. Elsevier
4. Altfeld M, Fadda L, Frleta D, Bhardwaj N (2011) DCs and NK cells: critical effectors in the immune response to HIV-1. Nat Rev Immunol 11:176–186
5. Slamon DJ, Leyland-Jones B, Shak S, Fuchs H, Paton V, Bajamonde A, Fleming T, Eiermann W, Wolter J, Pegram M, Baselga J, Norton L (2001) Use of chemotherapy plus a monoclonal antibody against HER2 for metastatic breast Cancer that overexpresses HER2. N Engl J Med 344(11):783–792. https://doi.org/10.1056/nejm200103153441101
6. Yu L, Wang Y, Yao Y, Li W, Lai Q, Li J, Zhou Y, Kang T, Xie Y, Wu Y, Chen X, Yi C, Gou L, Yang J (2014) Eradication of growth of HER2-positive ovarian cancer with trastuzumab-DM1, an antibody-cytotoxic drug conjugate in mouse xenograft model. Int J Gynecol Cancer 24(7):1158–1164. https://doi.org/10.1097/igc.0000000000000179
7. Tak W, Mak MES (2006) MHC: the major histocompatibility complex. The immune response. Elsevier
8. Brunner KT, Mauel J, Cerottini JC, Chapuis B (1968) Quantitative assay of the lytic action of immune lymphoid cells on 51-Cr-labelled allogeneic target cells in vitro; inhibition by isoantibody and by drugs. Immunology 14 (2):181–196
9. Kiessling R, Klein E (1973) Cytotoxic potential of mouse spleen cells on H-2 antibody-treated target cells. J Exp Med 137 (2):527–532
10. Zaritskaya L, Shurin MR, Sayers TJ, Malyguine AM (2010) New flow cytometric assays for monitoring cell-mediated cytotoxicity. Expert Rev Vaccines 9(6):601–616. https://doi.org/10.1586/erv.10.49
11. NK cell isolation kit. Miltenyi Biotec. http://www.miltenyibiotec.com/en/products-and-services/macs-cell-separation/cell-separation-reagents/microbeads-and-isolation-kits/nk-cells/nk-cell-isolation-kit-human.aspx
12. CellTrace™ CFSE Cell Proliferation Kit, for flow cytometry. ThermoFisher Scientific. https://www.thermofisher.com/order/catalog/product/C34554

Part III

Animal Models

Chapter 14

Evaluation of Breast Cancer and Melanoma Metastasis in Syngeneic Mouse Models

Kristina Witt and Andreas Lundqvist

Abstract

Syngeneic mouse models enable us to study the interaction of the immune system with tumor cells during tumor development and metastasis. It further allows us to evaluate the efficacy of immunotherapies on the different stages of tumor growth and the metastatic process. Here we describe two syngeneic mouse models, a murine mammary carcinoma and a murine melanoma model, that are used to study metastasis. Metastases occur spontaneously in the murine mammary carcinoma. The presence and number of foci are evaluated by culturing the lung tissue in a colony formation assay. For the murine melanoma model, tumor cells are injected intravenously, and metastatic burden is analyzed by counting of metastatic lesions.

Key words Syngeneic mouse model, Murine mammary carcinoma, Murine melanoma, 4T1 cell line, B16F10 cell line, Metastasis, Spontaneous metastasis

1 Introduction

With the great interest in developing new immunotherapies for cancer therapy, there is a growing need to understand the interaction between immune cells and tumors in more depth. It is now established knowledge that immune cells are in close contact with tumor cells. In early tumor development, the immune system is directed against the malignant tumor cells and able to eliminate those. However, over time and under the pressure of the immune system, tumor cells escape the antitumor-directed immune response [1]. They acquire mechanisms to avoid recognition by immune cells and induce suppressive immune cells. It becomes quite clear that treatments targeting the immune system should be tailored to the immune status of the patient.

Immunotherapy has also been shown to be especially potent targeting metastasis [2]. Mouse models that enable to not only study tumor development and growth but also the metastatic process and burden are therefore valuable tools for the development of immunotherapies.

Yago Pico de Coaña (ed.), *Immune Checkpoint Blockade: Methods and Protocols*, Methods in Molecular Biology, vol. 1913, https://doi.org/10.1007/978-1-4939-8979-9_14, © Springer Science+Business Media, LLC, part of Springer Nature 2019

Syngeneic mouse models enable us to study the coevolution of tumor and immune cells in vivo as well as the interplay of immune cells. The syngeneic mouse models are based on the establishment of murine tumor cell lines that can be inoculated into immunocompetent mice of the strain they are derived from. In this protocol we have focused on the 4T1 and intravenous (i.v.) B16F10 model. They are of particular interest when studying the targeting of tumor metastasis using immunotherapy.

The 4T1 model is a spontaneous breast cancer model that closely mimics triple-negative breast cancer [3]. For the 4T1 model, the murine mammary carcinoma cell line 4T1 is inoculated orthotopically into the mammary fat pad. Three weeks after the inoculation, the primary tumors are harvested, and the lungs are processed to evaluate metastatic burden. The i.v. B16F10 model is based on the intravenous injection of the murine metastatic melanoma cell line B16F10. Upon injection the tumor cells establish small tumors in the lung, similar to metastasis derived from a primary tumor. The advantage of this model is that it is rather fast compared to other metastasis models. The tumor foci can be visually distinct from healthy tissue due to their black color and can therefore be easily enumerated. No further assays or analysis is required for the evaluation of the metastatic burden.

Both the 4T1 and the B16F10 models are commonly used in the development of novel immunotherapies and tumor immunology research.

2 Materials

2.1 4T1 Orthotopic Mammary Carcinoma Model

1. RPMI01640 medium.
2. FBS.
3. BALB/c mice, female.
4. 4T1 cell line.
5. Hair removal cream.
6. Isoflurane.
7. Vaporizer with facial mask.
8. 27G needle.
9. 1 ml syringe.
10. 70 % ethanol.
11. Caliper.
12. Ear puncher.
13. PBS.
14. PBS + 10% FBS.
15. Surgical tools.

16. Pins.
17. Cork board.
18. Tissues.
19. Ice.
20. 15 ml Falcon tubes.
21. 50 ml Falcon tubes.
22. 6-well plate.
23. Dissociation buffer: RPMI 1640 supplemented with 5% FBS, 2 mg/ml dispase, 100 μg/ml DNaseI, 200 μg/ml collagenase IV.
24. Scalpels.
25. ACK lysis buffer.
26. Selection medium: RPMI 1640, 10% FBS, 60 μM 6-thioguanine.
27. Tissue culture dish, 15 cm diameter with grid.
28. 4% formaldehyde.
29. Hematoxylin.
30. Heating lamp.

2.2 B16F10 i.v. Challenge

1. B16F10.
2. FBS.
3. PBS.
4. C57Bl/6, female.
5. Fekete solution: 580 ml 95% ethanol, 200 ml H_2O, 80 ml 37% formaldehyde solution, 40 ml glacial acetic acid; add ddH_2O up to 1 l.
6. 27G needle.
7. 70% ethanol.
8. 15 ml Falcon tube.
9. 50 ml Falcon tube.
10. 0.05% trypsin-EDTA.
11. Surgical tools.
12. Corkboard.
13. Pins.
14. Tissue.
15. Petri dish.
16. Heating lamp.

3 Methods

3.1 4T1 Orthotopic Breast Cancer Model

1. Use only age-matched female BALB/c mice for injection (*see* **Note 1**).
2. Remove fur around the fourth mammary ducts 1 day before tumor inoculation. Pick up each mouse individually and hold it on the scruff. Apply a thin layer of hair removal cream on the fur around the fourth mammary ducts (*see* **Note 2**).
3. Put mouse into empty cage. After 3 min of incubation, pick up mouse again and remove cream with a wetted paper towel (*see* **Note 3**). If hair removal was not completed, repeat Subheading 3.1, **steps 1** and **3**.
4. Culture 4T1 cell line in RPMI-1640 medium supplemented with 10% FBS. Grow cells to 70–80% confluency in culture flasks and harvest on injection day (*see* **Note 4**).
5. Remove cell culture medium and wash cells with PBS. To detach cells, add 0.05% trypsin-EDTA and incubate for 3 min at 37°C. Stop reaction with RPMI-1640 medium supplemented with 10% FBS. Transfer cells into 50 ml Falcon tube and wash cells twice with PBS. Resuspend cells in PBS and count. Adjust cell suspension to 4×10^6 cells/ml in PBS (*see* **Note 5**). Store cells on ice until injection (*see* **Note 6**).
6. Bring cells to animal facility and prepare mice for injection.
7. Anesthetize mice with 4% isoflurane, and keep anesthetized during injection using a face mask connected to a vaporizer (*see* **Note 7**).
8. Position mouse on the back; the abdomen should be facing toward you during injection.
9. Mix cell suspension by inverting the Falcon tube several times. Take up cell suspension for one mouse at a time, 50 μl, and attach 27G needle (*see* **Note 8**).
10. Disinfect injection site with tissue dipped in 70% ethanol.
11. Take duct in between the thumb and index finger, with ductal opening on the top, and lift gently up. Insert needle right under the ductal opening (*see* **Note 9**). Slowly insert 50 μl of cell suspension. Hold needle in position for 2 s after injection, and then slowly remove the needle (*see* **Note 10**).
12. If required, earmark mouse and place under heating lamp during wake-up phase. Control that motoric functions are okay (*see* **Note 11**).
13. Palp tumors twice per week measuring width, length, and height (*see* **Note 12**).
14. First tumors appear approximately 1 week after injection. Around 3 weeks tumors reach 1 cm^3 in size, time point to euthanize mice and evaluate lung metastatic burden (*see* **Note 13**).

15. Prepare 15 ml Falcon tubes with PBS to collect primary tumors in. Prepare 15 ml Falcon tubes with PBS + 10% FBS to collect lungs in.
16. Euthanize mice by CO_2 asphyxiation.
17. Fixate mice, abdominal site facing up, with pins on corkboard covered with tissue.
18. Primary tumors are located under the skin and can be easily cut out with surgical tools. Afterward remove as much skin as possible from the tumor (*see* **Note 14**). Weigh each tumor and transfer tumor into prepared Falcon tube (*see* **Note 15**). Store one ice.
19. For long time storage, tumors should be snap frozen in liquid nitrogen or embedded in OCT for immune fluorescence and IHC stainings. Tumors should be stored at −80°C.
20. To dissect lungs, set vertical cut on the thorax. Set an orthogonal cut underneath the rib cage. Flip skin laps up toward the axilla. Place a v-shaped cut from the sternum to the axilla through the rib cage (*see* **Note 16**). Lift up rib cage at the xiphoid cartilage, the end of sternum. The lungs are now exposed.
21. Lift up the trachea lightly with forceps and cut right above forceps (side of head) (*see* **Note 17**). The lung can now be removed from the thorax. Rinse lung in PBS. Transfer lungs directly into collection tubes and store on ice (*see* **Note 18**).
22. Transfer one lung at a time into a well of a 6-well plate and add 3 ml dissociation buffer. Use scalpels to dissect the lung into small pieces, as small as possible (*see* **Note 19**).
23. Process up to five lungs in parallel.
24. Incubate lungs for 20–30 min at 37 °C to start tissue digestion. Then start over at **step 22** with the next lungs.
25. Homogenize lung tissue by drawing and releasing tissue pieces into a 1 ml syringe without needle; repeat this **step 5** times (*see* **Note 20**).
26. Filter the cell suspension through a 70 μm filter and collect in 50 ml tube. Wash filter with 10 ml PBS. Centrifuge for 10 min at 250 × *g* at 4 °C.
27. Discard supernatants carefully and resuspend pellets in 2 ml red blood cell lysis buffer. Incubate for 3 min at RT. Stop reaction by adding 28 ml PBS + 2% FBS. Centrifuge for 10 min at 250 × *g* at 4 °C (*see* **Note 21**).
28. Resuspend pellets in 10 ml PBS + 2% FBS and filter through 40 μm filter. Collect flow through in a new 50 ml tube. Centrifuge for 10 min at 250 × *g* at 4 °C.
29. Resuspend cells in 20 ml selection medium and plate in culture dish, 15 cm diameter. Culture cells in 37 °C.
30. Continue with the next lungs at **step 22**.

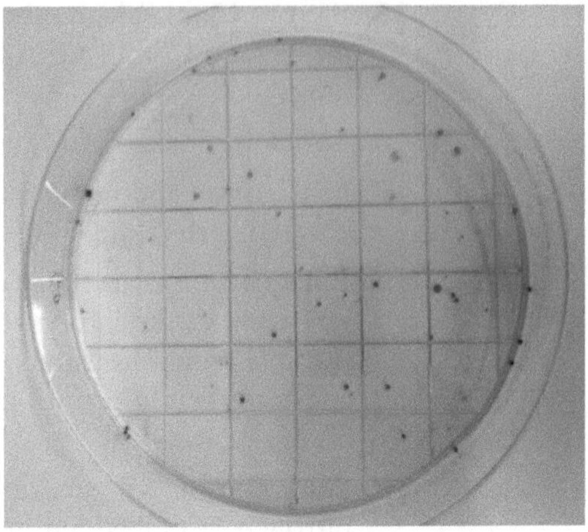

Fig. 1 Representative photo of colonies in colony formation assay

31. Change selection medium carefully every 3–4 days (*see* **Note 22**).
32. When colonies have become visible, remove medium on all plates. Wash plates with PBS.
33. Add 15 ml of 4% formaldehyde and incubate for 20 min at RT.
34. Take off the 4% formaldehyde and wash plates with water once (*see* **Note 23**).
35. Add 10 ml of hematoxylin and incubate for 10 min at RT.
36. Collect hematoxylin and wash twice with water (*see* **Note 24**).
37. Dry plates upside down on tissues overnight.
38. Enumerate number of colonies on each plate by manual counting. Divide colony number by tumor weight to get metastatic index (*see* **Note 25**) (Fig. 1).

3.2 B16F10 Intraveneous Metastasis Assay

1. Female C57Bl/6 mice in the age of 8–12 weeks are used for this assay (*see* **Note 26**).
2. Culture B16F10 cells in RPMI-1640 medium supplemented with 10% FBS. Grow B16F10 cells to 70–80% confluency (*see* **Note 4**).
3. Detach cells with 0.05% trypsin-EDTA for 3 min. Stop reaction with RPMI-1640 medium supplemented with 10% FBS. Wash cells twice with PBS. Count cells and resuspend to 2×10^6 cells/ml in PBS; keep in 50 ml tube. Keep cells on ice until injection (*see* **Note 5**).
4. Position heating lamp over cage to warm up mice (*see* **Note 27**).
5. Mix cell suspension by inverting several times. Take up cell suspension into syringe and attach 27G needle for one mouse at a time (*see* **Note 8**).

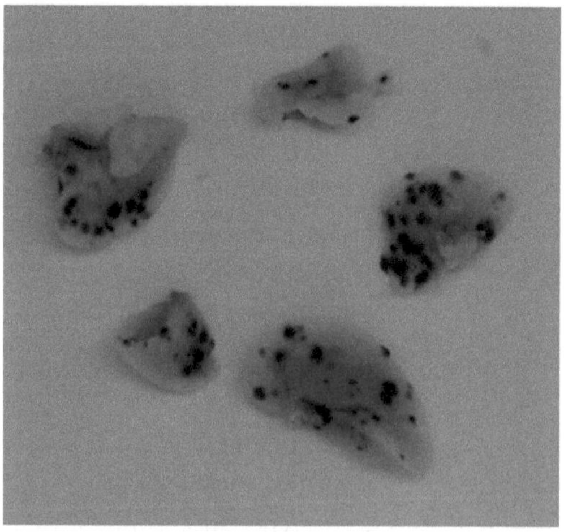

Fig. 2 Representative photo of lung metastases

6. Disinfect tail with tissue soaked in 70% ethanol.
7. Take one mouse at a time and place in restrainer (*see* **Note 28**).
8. Inject 100 μl of cell suspension into tail vein. Slowly withdraw needle from tail vein (*see* **Note 29**).
9. Take mouse out of restrainer.
10. Earmark mouse if required and place back in cage.
11. Euthanize mice by CO_2 asphyxiation.
12. Prepare 15 ml tubes with 5 ml Fekete solution for each lung.
13. Fixate mouse, abdominal site facing up, with pins on corkboard covered with tissue.
14. To dissect lungs, set vertical cut on the thorax. Set an orthogonal cut underneath the ribcage. Flip skin laps up toward the axilla. Place a v-shaped cut from the sternum to the axilla through the rib cage (*see* **Note 16**). Lift up ribcage at the xiphoid cartilage, the end of sternum. The lungs are now exposed.
15. Lift up the trachea lightly with forceps and cut right above forceps (side of head) (*see* **Note 17**). The lung can now be removed from the thorax. Rinse lungs in PBS. Transfer lungs directly into collection tubes and store on ice.
16. Transfer the lung into tube prepared with Fekete solution.
17. After overnight fixation (*see* **Note 30**), transfer the lung into petri dish. Separate lung lobes and enumerate foci for each lobe individually. Sum up the number of foci from all lobes to get the total number of foci in the lung per mouse (*see* **Notes 31** and **32**) (Fig. 2).
18. Keep a number of indicator mice in each experiment to monitor the size and number of lung metastasis (*see* **Note 28**).

4 Notes

1. Age match all mice to ensure reproducibility of data. It is advised to have 8–10 mice per group due to greater inter-mouse variance in this tumor model.
2. Hair removal cream has given the best results for fur removal around the ducts. Be advised to follow the application instructions given by the product regarding incubation time.
3. Wet tissue with 25–30 °C warm water to reduce stress for the mice due to cold temperature.
4. Tumor cells have to be in logarithmic growth phase prior to tumor inoculation.
5. Prepare three times as many cells than required for the injection to ensure that enough cells are available.
6. Keep time between harvest and injection as short as possible. Mix cell suspension from time to time to avoid clumping of the cells.
7. Keep mice no longer than 5 min under anesthesia. Mice cannot keep their temperature up during anesthesia. Therefore avoid placing mice onto metal surfaces during the procedure. Place them onto plastic surface covered with tissues.
8. Ensure that cells are well mixed before they are drawn into syringe. Take up twice as much volume of cell suspension into syringe. During the injection, the syringe should not be emptied completely. Cells tend to accumulate close to the plunger resulting in a more concentrated cell suspension in the end. Taking up the double volume prevents this.
9. Duct opening appears as a smart dot and should be the highest point during the injection. During the needle insertion, one can feel the needle tip in between the fingers. Insertion should be done approximately 2 mm under the duct opening.
10. Needle should be kept steady for a few seconds after the insertion of the suspension. This reduces the risk of leakage out of the injection site.
11. It is very important to check the motoric function after anesthesia to exclude that the anesthesia has impacted the neuronal function.
12. For tumors below a size of 1 mm^3, no precise measurement can be performed. Not down as present yes or no. Toward the end of the experiments, tumor can be ulcerating.
13. Lung metastasis can be visible as tiny dots; however it is not possible to see all micrometastasis and evaluate them visually.

14. The skin covers tumor and can easily be removed by pulling it off using forceps.
15. Tumor weight will be in the mg range. It is advised to use a scale in the mg range to note down as many differences as possible.
16. Do not cut into the lungs when cutting through the ribs.
17. The large vessel runs right next to the trachea. Avoid damaging this vessel to avoid contamination of the lung with blood. If this happens, rinse lungs with excessive lung to clean it.
18. It is possible that not all lung lobes are removed in one go. This is not of greater concern as long as all lobes are harvested and processed together later on. Each lung consists of five lobes in total.
19. Work as fast as possible once the first lung is in association buffer. One should avoid difference in incubation times between the different lungs to keep conditions as similar as possible. It is preferential to keep cells on ice than to process more to many lungs in parallel.
20. Splashes can occur when big pieces are drawn into syringe or let out. Work slowly to reduce the risk of splashes. The smaller the pieces, the better it is.
21. Repeat Subheading 3.1, **step 26** if red blood cell lysis was not complete.
22. Carefully tilt the culture plate and slowly take out medium without creating too much draft. Then add fresh conditioned medium slowly.
23. Collect washing liquids together with formaldehyde solution for correct disposal.
24. Hematoxylin can be reused twice. Make sure that washing liquids are collected together with hematoxylin for correct disposal.
25. Always normalize the number of metastasis to the primary tumor weight. In this model larger tumors metastasize more than smaller tumors. Interventions that would result in changes of primary tumor sizes have a direct influence on the metastatic burden of the lung.
26. Female mice are preferentially used due to easier handling.
27. Warm up animals prior to injection to enlarge the vessels. Work fast once the mouse is in the restrainer to prevent cooling down of the mouse. If tail veins still appear small, exposing the tail directly for 1 min to heat will enlarge them.
28. Position the mouse in a restrainer. It does not harm or hurt them. It reduces their movement and enables you to have two hands free for the injection.

29. Tail vein injections require practice and especially in the C57Bl/6 mice are the veins difficult to be seen. Practice the injection technique with PBS prior to this experiment. Set first injection at the far end of the tail. In the case that insertion into the vein did not succeed, the injection may be performed at a location on the tail closer to the body. If cells were injected by mistake into the tail and not the vein, remove this animal out of the experiment.
30. Lungs can be stored for long time after fixation. Take fixed lung out of Fekete solution, and store dry in a tightly closed vial at RT.
31. Blind lungs prior to enumeration to avoid bias as much as possible.
32. Indicator mice enable you to determine the optimal time point for the experimental endpoint. Metastasis burden can vary in between different experiments and responsible scientists.

References

1. Dunn GP, Old LJ, Schreiber RD (2004) The three Es of cancer immunoediting. Annu Rev Immunol 22:329–360. https://doi.org/10.1146/annurev.immunol.22.012703.104803
2. Turcotte S, Rosenberg SA (2011) Immunotherapy for metastatic solid cancers. Adv Surg 45:341–360
3. Kaur P, Nagaraja GM, Zheng H, Gizachew D, Galukande M, Krishnan S, Asea A (2012) A mouse model for triple-negative breast cancer tumor-initiating cells (TNBC-TICs) exhibits similar aggressive phenotype to the human disease. BMC Cancer 12:120. https://doi.org/10.1186/1471-2407-12-120

Chapter 15

Establishment of Melanoma Tumor Xenograft Using Single Cell Line Suspension and Co-injection of Patient-Derived T Cells in Immune-Deficient NSG Mice

Fríða Björk Gunnarsdóttir, Rolf Kiessling, and Yago Pico de Coaña

Abstract

When primary tumor cells are grown in vitro, they are exposed to an environment that is vastly different from the tumor environment they originate from. The in vitro environment can lack the three-dimensional structure of the tumor, other cell types present within the tumor microenvironment, and important growth factors. Humanized mouse models allow researchers to study primary tumor cells in a more natural environment. With further development of several strains of immune-deficient mice, the mouse model allows for observation of the patient-derived tumor xenograft (PDTX) growth alone as well as in the presence of a human immune system. We describe how this can be accomplished with injection of single cell suspension of melanoma tumor cells into immune-deficient NOD-scid IL2Rγ^{null} (NSG) mice. We also describe how tumor cells and immune cells can be co-injected, using Winn assay, and the possibility to use that method to study immune therapies for cancer.

Key words Xenograft, NSG mice, Melanoma, Immune deficiency, Tumor-infiltrating lymphocytes

1 Introduction

Even though in vitro experiments allow for exploration of pathways and interactions in immunology, they do not provide the same accuracy as in vivo studies. In vitro experiments lack the necessary cell-cell interaction and three-dimensional structure found in the human body [1]. Therefore, it is common to use animal models to perform in vivo experiments. The most common animal model is the murine model, or mouse model. Mice are easy to breed and handle, have a short generation time and accelerated life span compared to humans. Mice are mammals and relatively related to humans, their genome has been sequenced, and many different strains with genetic mutations are commercially available [2].

Mouse models are valuable for obtaining in vivo results, but there are some limitations that must be addressed. The most obvious limitation is that mice are not the same species as humans and

Yago Pico de Coaña (ed.), *Immune Checkpoint Blockade: Methods and Protocols*, Methods in Molecular Biology, vol. 1913, https://doi.org/10.1007/978-1-4939-8979-9_15, © Springer Science+Business Media, LLC, part of Springer Nature 2019

Table 1
Common immune-deficient mouse models and their phenotype

Mouse strain	Phenotype	Ref.
Athymic *Foxn1*^{nu} (nude)	Lacks T cells	[10]
C.B17-*Prkdc*^{scid} (*scid*)	Lacks mature T and B cells	[11, 12]
NOD.C.B17-*Prkdc*^{scid} (NOD-*scid*)	Lacks mature T and B cells, has decreased innate immunity with functionally immature macrophages and low NK cell function	[13]
NOD-*Prkdc*^{scid} *IL2rg*^{null} (NSG)	Lacks mature T and B cells, no NK cells and further impaired innate immunity due to defect of the high affinity receptor and no signaling through multiple cytokine receptors	[14, 15]

their immune system spontaneously rejects human tumors, so syngeneic models should be used. If focus is to be set on the growth of human tumors in vivo, immune-deficient mouse models are commonly used [3]. The most frequent ones can be seen in Table 1 where the phenotype of each strain, in regard to the immune response, is listed.

In tumor immunology, it is important to be able to look at the interaction between patient's immune system and malignant cells. By transplanting tumor cells or tissue into NSG mice, a patient-derived xenograft (PDX) can be created. This can be accomplished by either implanting whole tumor pieces or a single cell suspension of tumor cells subcutaneously or into specific organs [4]. With NSG mice being severely deficient in innate immunity as well as being completely deficient in adaptive immunity, they serve as an optimal PDX mouse model [2].

Along with tumor xenograft, immune cells can also be transplanted, humanizing both the tumor and immune system of PDX mice. In this setting, studies on the interaction between the human immune system and compatible tumor can be performed. These experiments can be done by using donor-unrelated human hematopoietic stem cells (HSCs) that develop into mature immune cells or by using peripheral blood mononuclear cells (PBMCs), but both of these options have limitations, including the development of graft-versus-host disease (GVHD) [5]. Another approach would be to co-engraft donor-matched tumors and immune cells limiting the chance for GVHD [6]. This can be done using Winn assay where patient-derived tumor cells and lymphoid cells from the same patient are mixed and simultaneously injected into NSG mice [7]. This method can be used to study the ability of the immune system to locally limit tumor growth and to evaluate the efficacy of immunotherapeutic approaches such as checkpoint blockade or adoptive cell transfer.

In this chapter, we will describe a method to establish melanoma PDX in NSG mice from a single cell suspension of tumor cells. We also describe establishment of a PDX using a Winn assay.

2 Materials

Make sure all equipment is sterile. Wipe down all surfaces before starting the experiment.

2.1 Tumor Acquisition and Preparation

1. Scalpel.
2. Tweezers: either metal or plastic sterile tweezers.
3. Petri dish or a 6-well cell culture plate.
4. PBS: 1× phosphate-buffered saline solution.
5. 1 mL pipette and tips
6. Eppendorf tubes.
7. Cell strainer: 40 μm nylon strainer that fits onto the top of a 50 mL Falcon tube.
8. 50 mL Falcon tube
9. Grinder (*see* **Note 1**).

2.2 Patient-Derived Melanoma Xenograft

1. 0.4% trypan blue.
2. Hemocytometer.
3. Mice (*see* **Note 2**).
4. PBS: 1× phosphate-buffered saline solution.
5. Eppendorf tubes.
6. 1 mL syringe
7. Needle: Gauge <25 g.
8. Caliper.

2.3 Tumor Passage

1. Scalpel.
2. Tweezers.
3. Surgical scissors.
4. Petri dish.
5. PBS: 1× phosphate-buffered saline solution.
6. Cell strainer: 40 μm nylon strainer that fits onto the top of a 50 mL Falcon tube.
7. 50 mL Falcon tube
8. Grinder (*see* **Note 1**).
9. 0.4% trypan blue.
10. Hemocytometer.
11. Mice (*see* **Note 2**).

12. 1 mL syringe
13. Needle: Gauge <25 g.

2.4 Winn Assay

1. Tumor-infiltrating lymphocyte suspension of appropriate concentration (*see* **Note 3**).
2. Tumor single cell suspension.
3. PBS: 1× phosphate-buffered saline solution.
4. Eppendorf tubes.
5. 1 mL syringe
6. Needle: Gauge <25 g.

3 Methods

Carry out all experiments under sterile conditions, in a flow cabinet, in order to prevent contamination of samples. Work as fast as possible to keep samples fresh and store samples on ice after preparation and during transportation.

3.1 Tumor Acquisition and Preparation

1. After surgical removal of melanoma tumor from patient, transfer tumor in liquid, preferably 20% RPMI medium or PBS. Start the single cell suspension protocol immediately after tumor acquisition to limit cell death.
2. Place tumor into a petri dish or well in a 6-well plate with PBS. Using scalpels and sterilized tweezers, cut the tumor into fragments, as small as possible.
3. Transfer tumor fragments and PBS with a 25 or 50 mL pipette onto a cell strainer on top of a 50 mL Falcon tube.
4. Grind tumor pieces through strainer and wash strainer every now and then with PBS. Fill tube to 50 mL with PBS.
5. Spin down the single cell suspension, resuspend, and count cells.
6. Single cell suspension can be used to establish a tumor cell line as well as establish a primary melanoma xenograft in mice.
7. Leftover single cell suspension can be spun down, resuspended in freezing media, and kept frozen at −80 °C for later use.

3.2 Primary Melanoma Xenograft

The single cell suspension can be used to establish primary melanoma xenografts in mouse models. Make sure to keep samples on ice during transportation and preparation in animal facility. Always wear protective gloves when handling NSG mice, and work under sterile conditions to avoid infecting the mice.

1. Dilute single cell suspension with PBS to desired concentration (*see* **Notes 3** and **4**). Transfer to a sterile Eppendorf tube and keep on ice until injected into mice.

2. Prepare the syringe by placing the needle on the syringe. Line the bevel with the numbers on the syringe so you can monitor the injected volume while you inject.
3. Slowly pull up 200 μl of cell suspension. Make sure to get rid of all bubbles in the syringe before injection, holding the syringe vertical, flicking it, and pushing out the air until liquid comes out of the needle. Always prepare your syringe before restraining the mouse.
4. Restrain the mouse, either physically or with chemical restraint such as gas anesthesia (*see* **Note 5**). If you are using physical restraint, use your non-dominant hand to restrain so your dominant hand is free for the injection. Try to limit the restraining time to minimize discomfort to the animal.
5. Inject the single cell suspension subcutaneously into right or left flank of the mouse. While holding the needle parallel to the abdomen, pierce the skin of flank, with the bevel side of the needle facing up. Take care to only pierce the skin and not the fat layer under the skin, avoiding injection into internal organs or abdominal cavity.
6. Inject 200 μl of cell suspension slowly but steady into either the left or right flank of the mouse (*see* **Note 6**). A new needle should be used for each mouse inoculated.
7. After injection, monitor mice regularly and measure tumor growth. Tumor growth is measured by palping the mice, feeling the flank for tumors, and measuring the width, length, and height or depth of the tumor in mm using a caliper.
8. Replace animal back to cage and observe for any complications.
9. When tumor reaches maximum size in mm^3 allowed by the ethical permit, it can be excised and used to prepare a single cell suspension for passage into additional mice.

3.3 Tumor Passage

Always wear protective gloves when handling NSG mice, and work under sterile conditions to avoid infecting the mice.

1. When tumors have reached maximum size allowed by the ethical permit, the mice should be euthanized (*see* **Note** 7).
2. After euthanasia, place the mouse on its back and wet the fur of the injection site with ethanol. This is to minimize fur contamination of the tumor excised.
3. With surgical scissors cut the skin over the tumor carefully, taking care not to puncture the tumor mass.
4. With tweezers and scalpel, remove the tumor, preferably in one piece, and move to a petri dish (*see* **Note 8**).
5. Wash the tumor with PBS and then move to another clean petri dish.

6. Cut the tumor into small fragments using scalpel, and move the tumor pieces and PBS from petri dish to a cell strainer on top of a 50 mL Falcon tube. Grind tumor using same method as described above.
7. Inject the single cell suspension subcutaneously into right or left flank of the new NSG mice (*see* **Note 9**).

3.4 Winn Assay

Make sure to work under sterile conditions to avoid contamination of samples. Always wear protective gloves when working with samples and NSG mice. Keep samples on ice while working with them and for transportation.

1. Determine cell concentration of TIL suspension and tumor single cell suspension. Adjust to desired cell concentration (*see* **Note 3**).
2. Transfer samples to animal house, and prepare everything needed to conduct the Winn assay *BEFORE* mixing the two cell suspensions, including animals and syringe.
3. In an Eppendorf tube, mix TIL suspension and tumor single cell suspension in desired ratio.
4. Immediately draw 200 μl of cell suspension into the syringe. Make sure to get rid of all bubbles in the syringe before injection, holding the syringe vertical, flicking it, and pushing out the air until liquid comes out of the needle.
5. Inject the cell suspension subcutaneously into right or left flank of the mouse.
6. Evaluate tumor growth. If the TILs recognize the tumor cells, tumor growth is stalled or inhibited as can be seen in Fig. 1.

4 Notes

1. Grinders are available from many different companies and come in plastic, glass, and metal variations. The end of a 2 mL plastic syringe handle makes for a good grinder. It has a rough surface that is suitable for grinding tissue.
2. NSG mice are the most preferred model in this case due to their lack of adaptive immune cells and severely deficient innate immunity.
3. Cell number injected. We recommend starting injection number of 1×10^6 cells. This can vary between patients, with some aggressive melanoma needing fewer cells injected and some needing more. This calls for titration of the cells, and, as can be seen in Fig. 2, cell number injected can give variable results in tumor growth. Tumors have been successfully implanted in a murine model using only a single melanoma cell [8]. The same

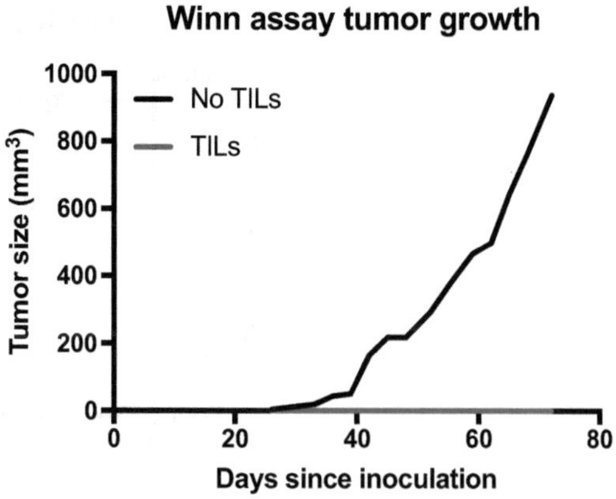

Fig. 1 Tumor growth of PDX melanoma tumor in NSG mice. Mice were either co-injected with a mixture of TILs and tumor cells in ratio 1:1 ($n = 2$) or tumor cells alone with PBS ($n = 2$). Mice co-injected with TILs and tumor cells show now tumor growth by day 72, while tumors in mice injected with tumor cells alone reach the maximum size of 1000 mm^3 by that time

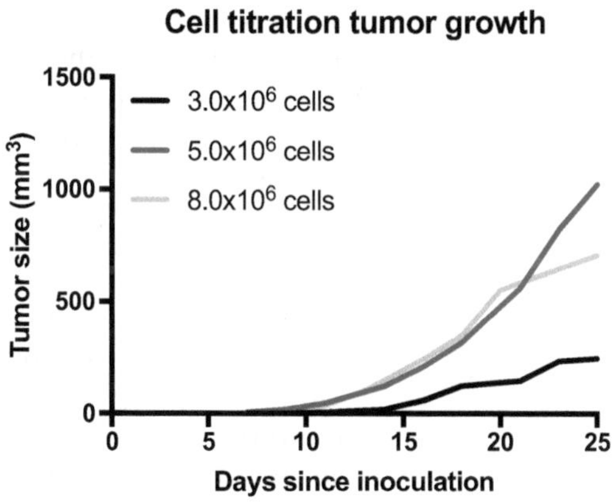

Fig. 2 Growth of PDX melanoma tumor in NSG mice. Mice were injected with three million cells ($n = 3$), five million cells ($n = 8$), or eight million cells ($n = 8$). All groups have palpable tumors by day 9, but mice injected with three million tumor cells have delayed tumor growth observed compared to mice injected with either five million or eight million tumor cells

goes for Winn assay where titration of both tumor cells and lymphoid cells is advised. The effect of different tumor/lymphoid cell ratios can be seen in Fig. 3.

4. Tumor cells can be co-injected with Matrigel. This can enhance the tumor growth by improving the attachment and differentiation of the cell and mimics the 3D environment. This can result in fewer cells needed to establish tumor growth in the murine model [9].

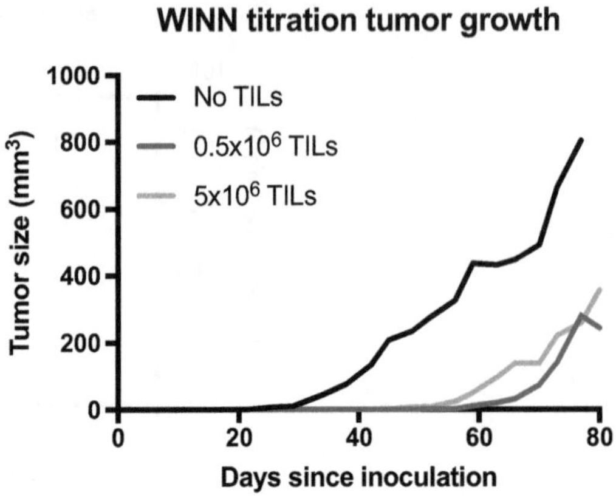

Fig. 3 Tumor growth of PDX melanoma tumor. 5×10^6 tumor cells were co-injected with patient-derived TILs, using Winn assay. Ratio injected (TILs/tumor cells) of 1:1 ($n = 3$) and 1:10 ($n = 3$). For negative control, PBS was used ($n = 3$). When mice were co-injected with tumor cells and TILs, a delayed tumor growth was observed for both ratios, compared to negative control

5. To physically restrain a mouse, it is best to grab the scruff of the mouse and secure the tail under either pinky or ring finger. Make sure the mouse is held firmly and that is unable to bite or move around. Then turn your hand, exposing the abdomen of the mouse.
6. Injection into the flank is not the most common location for subcutaneous injection into mouse models. The most common one is into the loose skin over the shoulders, the scruff. To inject into the scruff, hold the mouse face down, grab the scruff, and lift up the skin. Stick the needle into the scruff, toward the rear end of the mouse. Take care to only pierce the skin and not the fat layer under the skin.
7. Euthanasia of mice can be done with CO_2 gas, with decapitation, or with injectables. CO_2 should not be used as the sole means of euthanasia. It must be followed by a secondary method such as decapitation.
8. If excess skin is stuck to the tumor, try to remove as much as possible, using a scalpel to peel or shave the tumor loose from the skin.
9. With increased passage number, clonal selection of the tumor may occur. This can result in cells that are more efficient at establishing tumors to be selected for and will increase the growth rate of tumors in the mouse model as can be seen in Fig. 4. With higher passage number, the integrity of the xenograft tumor can be compromised. We recommend comparative genetic analysis of the original tumor with the subsequent passages.

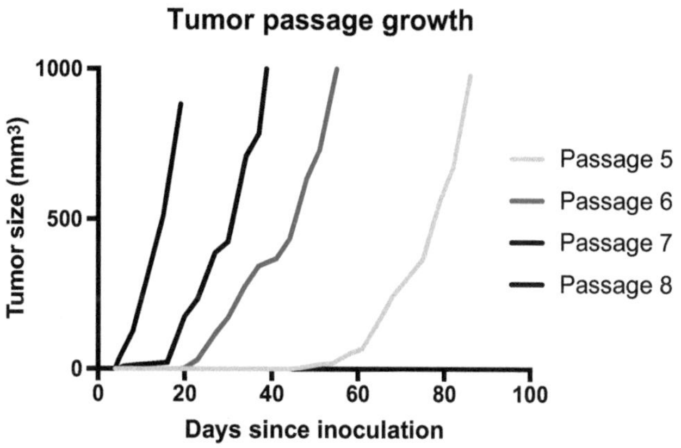

Fig. 4 Tumor growth of PDX melanoma tumor passage. Passage 5 ($n = 3$) is not palpable until day 44, while passage 6 ($n = 4$) is palpable already at day 20 in comparison. Later passages 7 ($n = 2$) and 8 ($n = 2$) are both palpable within 10 days. All passages show a similar growth curve. Through increased passages, tumor growth is increased, indicating clonal selection of the tumor cells

References

1. Morton JJ, Bird G, Refaeli Y, Jimeno A (2016) Humanized mouse xenograft models: narrowing the tumor-microenvironment gap. Cancer Res 76:6153–6158
2. Schultz LD, Goodwin N, Ishikawa F et al (2014) Human cancer growth and therapy in NOD/SCID/IL2Rγ^{null} (NSG) mice. Cold Spring Harb Protoc 7:694–708
3. Schultz LD, Ishikawa F, Greiner DL (2007) Humanized mice in translational biomedical research. Nat Rev Immunol 7:118–130
4. Jung J (2014) Human tumor xenograft models for preclinical assessment of anticancer drug development. Toxicol Res 30:1–5
5. Decker WK, da Silva RD, Sanabria MH et al (2017) Cancer immunotherapy: historical perspective of a clinical revolution and emerging preclinical animal models. Front Immunol 8:829
6. Simpson-Abelson MR, Sonnenberg GF, Takita H et al (2008) Long-term engraftment and expansion of tumor derived memory T cells following the implantation of non-disrupted pieces of human lung tumor into NOD-scid IL2Rγnull mice. J Immunol 180:7009–7018
7. Winn HJ (1961) Immune mechanisms in homotransplantation II. Quantitative assay of immunologic activity of lymphoid cells stimulated by tumor homografts. J Immunol 86:228–239
8. Quintana E, Shackleton M, Sabel MS et al (2008) Efficient tumor formation by single human melanoma cells. Nature 456:593–598
9. Kleinman HK, Martin GR (2005) Matrigel: basement membrane matrix with biological activity. Semin Cancer Biol 15(5):378–386
10. Fogh J, Fogh JM, Orfeo T (1977) One hundred and twenty-seven cultured human tumor cell lines producing tumors in nude mice. J Natl Cancer Inst 59:221–226
11. Bosma GC, Custer RP, Bosma MJ (1983) A severe combined immunodeficiency mutation in the mouse. Nature 301:527–530
12. Blunt T, Gell D, Fox M et al (1996) Identification of a nonsense mutation in the carboxyl-terminal region of DNA-dependent protein kinase catalytic subunit in the scid mouse. Proc Natl Acad Sci U S A 93:10285–10290
13. Schultz LD, Schweitzer PA, Christianson SW et al (1995) Multiple defects in innate and adaptive immunologic function on NOD/LtSz-scid mice. J Immunol 154:180–191
14. Cao X, Shores EW, Hu-Li J et al (1995) Defective lymphoid development in mice lacking expression of the common cytokine receptor gamma chain. Immunity 2:223–238
15. DiSanto JP, Muller W, Guy-Grand D, Fischer A, Rajewsky K (1995) Lymphoid development in mice with a targeted deletion of the interleukin 2 receptor gamma chain. Proc Natl Acad Sci U S A 92:377–381

Chapter 16

Analysis of Tissue-Resident Immune Cells from Mouse Skin and Lungs by Flow Cytometry

Felipe Galvez-Cancino, Ernesto Lopez, and Alvaro Lladser

Abstract

The heterogeneity and complexity of nonlymphoid tissues has become a major obstacle for the study of immune populations. For this reason, the generation of highly reproducible protocols that allow the analysis of immune cells in these tissues has become crucial for clinical and preclinical research. Here we describe an optimized method that allows the obtention of single-cell suspensions from the skin and lungs to analyze and quantify populations of tissue-resident memory CD8$^+$ T cells by multi-parametric flow cytometry.

Key words Flow cytometry, Barrier tissues, Immunophenotyping, Memory CD8$^+$ T cells, Single-cell suspensions

1 Introduction

The study of leukocytes has been classically focused on secondary lymphoid organs (SLO) such as the spleen and lymph nodes due to their high abundance and easy isolation [1]. However, the presence of lymphocytes that stably reside in nonlymphoid barrier tissues such as the skin, lung, gut, and female reproductive tract, as well as non-barrier tissues, including the brain, liver, and others, has attracted the attention of immunologists because they play a key role in maintaining tissue integrity and function during homeostasis and disease [2–4]. We have recently shown that skin vaccination induces the accumulation of tissue-resident memory CD8$^+$ T (Trm) cells in the skin but not in the lungs. These Trm cells were able to mediate strong protection against cutaneous melanoma in absence of other populations of circulating memory CD8$^+$ T cells [5].

Analysis of immune cell populations by flow cytometry allows the detection of several parameters including cell size, their complexity, and the presence of surface and intracellular proteins in

Yago Pico de Coaña (ed.), *Immune Checkpoint Blockade: Methods and Protocols*, Methods in Molecular Biology, vol. 1913, https://doi.org/10.1007/978-1-4939-8979-9_16, © Springer Science+Business Media, LLC, part of Springer Nature 2019

single-cell suspensions, becoming a crucial technique for clinical and preclinical research [6, 7].

Given the heterogeneity and complexity of nonlymphoid tissues, obtaining single-cell suspensions to be analyzed by flow cytometry represents a major challenge. Here, we describe an optimized methodology that allows the preparation and analysis by flow cytometry of single-cell suspensions obtained from the skin and lungs. These protocols have been used to characterize tissue-resident memory CD8$^+$ T cells in mice.

2 Materials

2.1 Enzymes

1. Collagenase D (Gibco, catalog number: 17104-019) 1000 U/mL.
2. DNase I (AppliChem, catalog number: 9003-98-9) grade II, 20 U/mL prepared in Hank's buffered saline solution (HBSS) without Ca^{+2} and Mg^{+2}.

2.2 Solutions

1. R10: RPMI + 10% FBS.
2. Stop buffer: R10 containing ethylenediaminetetraacetic acid (EDTA) 5 mM.
3. Red blood cell lysis buffer (BioLegend, catalog number 420301).
4. Phosphate-buffered saline (PBS).
5. TruStain fcX (anti-mouse CD16/32) antibody (BioLegend, catalog number 101320).
6. PBS-FBS 2%.

2.3 Other Materials

1. Microscope slides with ground edge.
2. 70 μm cell strainer.
3. Small and sharp scissors.
4. 24× well plate.
5. EDTA pH 8.0 0.5 M.

3 Methods

1. Carry out all procedures at room temperature unless otherwise specified.
2. Sacrifice the mouse using a CO_2 chamber (*see* **Note 1**).

   Lungs: Take the tissue avoiding taking pieces of the thymus, trachea, and heart.

   Back skin: Take 15–20 mg of shaved tissue (approximately 2 cm^2). Eliminate subcutaneous fat with scalpel avoiding to remove part of the dermis.

3. Place the tissue into a 24-well plate containing 895 μL of RPMI without supplements, and chop it with scissors into small pieces. Then, add 100 μL of collagenase D and 5 μL DNase I pre-warmed at 37 °C (*see* **Note 1**).
4. Incubate the plate containing the tissues:

   Lungs: 1 h at 37 °C with shaking.
   Skin: 30 min in a CO_2 incubator at 37 °C without shaking.
5. Add 1 mL of stop buffer to each well and pipet up and down several times to increase tissue disaggregation, mesh the tissue using microscope cover slides with ground edges, and filter through a 70 μm cell strainer into 15 mL conic tubes to obtain a single-cell suspension. Finally, wash the well, the microscope slides, and the cell strainer with 5 mL of R10 to allow remaining cells to pass through.
6. Centrifuge the tubes containing the cell suspension at 400 × *g* at 4 °C, for 5 min. Resuspend the cell pellet in 1 mL of R10 containing 25 μL of DNase and incubate 5 min on ice (*see* **Note 2**). If needed, filter the single-cell suspension through a 70 μm cell strainer to remove cell aggregates.
7. Centrifuge the tubes containing the cell suspension at 400 × *g*, 4 °C, for 5 min. Aspirate the supernatant and resuspend the cells in 100 μL TruStain fcX. Plate the 1–5 × 10^6 of cells in a 96-well round bottom plate and incubate 20 min at 4 °C without light (*see* **Note 3**).
8. Add 100 μL of PBS-FBS 2% and centrifuge the plate containing the cell suspension at 400 × *g*, 4 °C, for 5 min.
9. Prepare the following cocktail of antibodies to identify $CD8^+$ T cells (Table 1) (*see* **Note 4**).
10. Stain the cells by adding 30 μL of antibody cocktail per well at 4 °C during 20 min in darkness.
11. Wash the cells twice with 150 μL of PBS-FBS 2% centrifuging the plate at 900 × *g* for 2 min, and resuspend the cells in 150 μL of PBS-FBS 2%. Cells are ready to be analyzed by flow cytometry.
12. $CD8^+$ T cells in the skin and lungs of naïve mice are shown in Fig. 1. In both tissues 40–50% of the cells are dead. This is due to tissue disaggregation and enzymatic digestion. The frequencies of hematopoietic cells ($CD45^+$) found were 47.8% and 95.6% in the skin and lungs, respectively. Our protocol of cell extraction has been designed to enrich the immune cell compartment that together with the gating strategy allows to have high frequencies of $CD45^+$ cells.

Table 1
Antibody cocktail to identify CD8$^+$ T cells in the skin and lungs

Antibody	Fluorophore	Clone	Company	Dilution
CD45 (*see* **Note 4**)	PE	30-F11	BioLegend®	1/800
CD8	PE-Cy7	53–5.8	BioLegend®	1/250
CD3	Brilliant violet 421	17A2	BioLegend®	1/200
CD103	PerCP-Cy5.5	2E7	BioLegend®	1/200
CD69	APC	H1.2F3	BioLegend®	1/200
CD49a	APC	HMα1	BioLegend®	1/200
Zombie aqua	Brilliant violet 510		BioLegend®	1/125

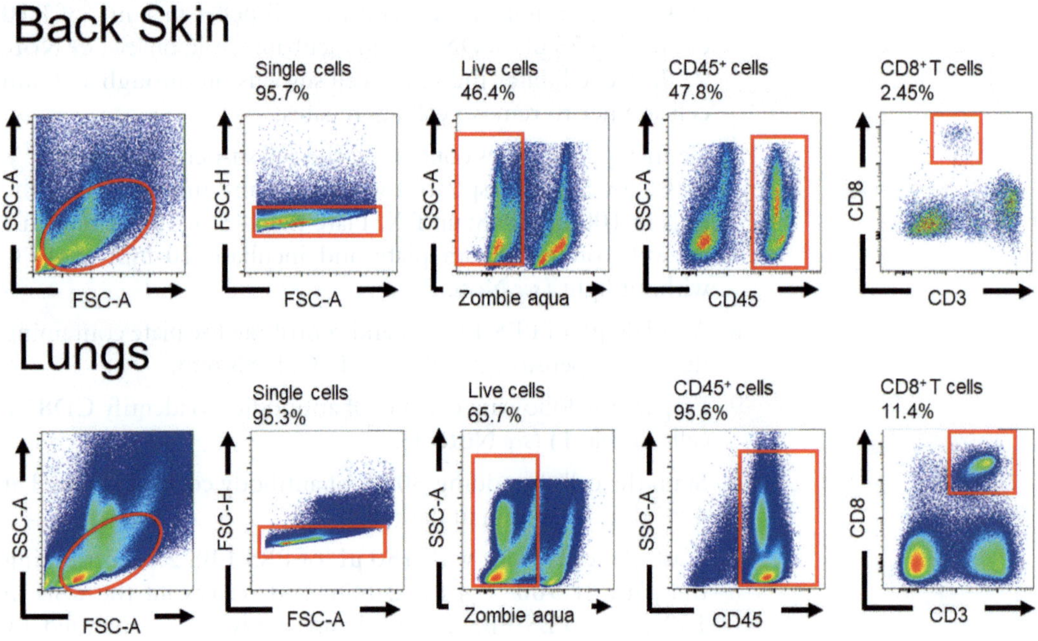

Fig. 1 CD8$^+$ T cell discrimination in the skin and lungs. The skin and lungs from naïve C57BL/6 mice were analyzed. Upper and lower panels show the gating strategy to identify CD8$^+$ T cells in the skin and in the lungs, respectively. Samples were acquired using the BD FACSCANTO™ II flow cytometer

13. Given our expertise working with tissue-resident memory CD8$^+$ T cells, we have focused on them as shown in Fig. 2 [5]. CD103, CD69, and CD49a define the tissue-resident memory T cell phenotype [8, 9]. As shown, most of the CD8$^+$ T cells display this phenotype in the skin, whereas CD8$^+$ T cells express lower levels of CD103, and there is no expression of CD69 and CD49a in lungs [10].

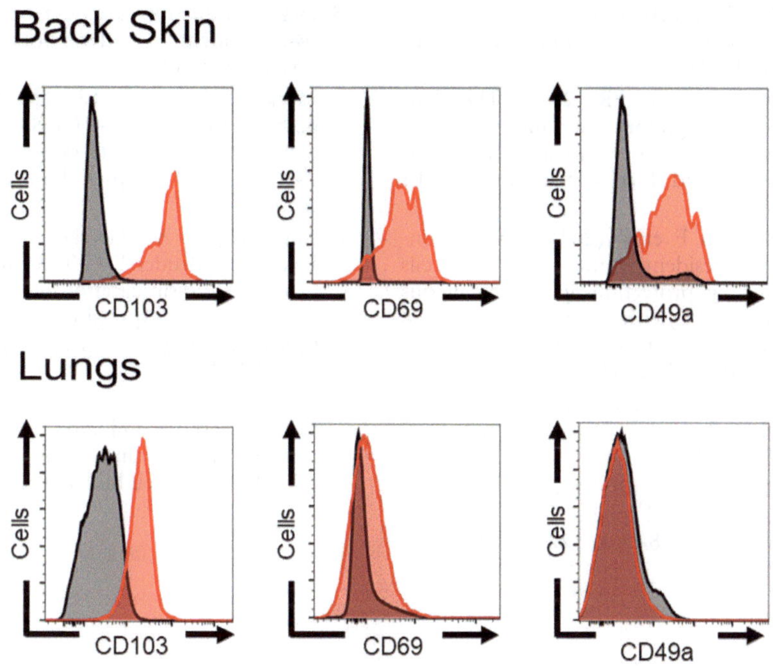

Fig. 2 Analysis of tissue-resident memory CD8$^+$ T cell markers in the skin and lungs. The skin and lungs from naïve C57BL/6 mice were analyzed. The expression of CD103, CD69, and CD49a was analyzed in total CD8$^+$ T cells from the skin (top panels) and lungs (bottom panels). Samples were acquired using the BD FACSCANTO™ II flow cytometer

4 Notes

1. Pre-warming the enzymes at 37 °C allows to have them at their maximum activity at the moment of starting tissue disaggregation.
2. Given the high amount of dead cells generated during tissue disaggregation, it is useful to make a second DNase digestion to eliminate DNA that can cause cell aggregation and clumping [11].
3. Antibody dilutions were set up to stain a maximum of 5×10^6 of cells.
4. Given the high amounts of stroma cells in the skin and in the lungs, CD45 staining allows to discard non-hematopoietic cells.

References

1. Steinert EM et al (2015) Quantifying memory CD8 T cells reveals regionalization of Immunosurveillance. Cell 161(4):737–749
2. Hooper LV, Littman DR, Macpherson AJ (2012) Interactions between the microbiota and the immune system. Science 336 (6086):1268–1273

3. Chen K, Kolls JK (2013) T cell-mediated host immune defenses in the lung. Annu Rev Immunol 31:605–633
4. Heath WR, Carbone FR (2013) The skin-resident and migratory immune system in steady state and memory: innate lymphocytes, dendritic cells and T cells. Nat Immunol 14 (10):978–985
5. Gálvez-Cancino F et al (2018) Vaccination-induced skin-resident memory CD8+ T cells mediate strong protection against cutaneous melanoma. OncoImmunology 7(7): e1442163. https://doi.org/10.1080/2162402x.2018.1442163
6. Fulwyler MJ (1965) Electronic separation of biological cells by volume. Science 150 (3698):910–911
7. Brown M, Wittwer C (2000) Flow cytometry: principles and clinical applications in hematology. Clin Chem 46(8 Pt 2):1221–1229
8. Fan X, Rudensky AY (2016) Hallmarks of tissue-resident lymphocytes. Cell 164:1198–1211
9. Mackay LK et al (2013) The developmental pathway for CD103(+)CD8+ tissue-resident memory T cells of skin. Nat Immunol 14:1294–1301. https://doi.org/10.1038/ni.2744
10. Autengruber A, Gereke M, Hansen G, Hennig C, Bruder D (2012) Impact of enzymatic tissue disintegration on the level of surface molecule expression and immune cell function. Eur J Microbiol Immunol (Bp) 2:112–120
11. Crissman HA, Mullaney PF, Steinkamp JA (1975) Methods and applications of flow systems for analysis and sorting of mammalian cells. Methods Cell Biol 9(0):179–246

Index

Yago Pico de Coaña (ed.), *Immune Checkpoint Blockade: Methods and Protocols*, Methods in Molecular Biology, vol. 1913, https://doi.org/10.1007/978-1-4939-8979-9, © Springer Science+Business Media, LLC, part of Springer Nature 2019

MIX
Papier aus verantwortungsvollen Quellen
Paper from responsible sources
FSC® C105338

If you have any concerns about our products,
you can contact us on
ProductSafety@springernature.com

In case Publisher is established outside the EU,
the EU authorized representative is:
Springer Nature Customer Service Center GmbH
Europaplatz 3, 69115 Heidelberg, Germany

Printed by Libri Plureos GmbH
in Hamburg, Germany